TX
392
.P53
1999

HWLCTC

Chicago Public Library
W9-BOC-284
Vegetables rock! : a complete guide

BUSINESS/SCIENCE/TECHNOLOGY DIVISION
CHICAGO PUBLIC LIBRARY
400 SOUTH STATE STREET
CHICAGO, IL 60605

Vegetables Rock!

BANTAM BOOKS

NEW YORK

TORONTO

LONDON

SYDNEY

AUCKLAND

Vegetables Rock!

A Complete Guide for Teenage Vegetarians

Stephanie Pierson

VEGETABLES ROCK!

A Bantam Book / March 1999

The vegetarian food pyramid is reprinted here courtesy of The Health Connection. It is available as a large poster, handout, and refrigerator magnet by calling 1-800-548-8700 or faxing 1-888-294-8405 for a free catalog.

All rights reserved.
Copyright © 1999 by Stephanie Pierson.
Cover art copyright © 1999 by Belina Huey.
BOOK DESIGN BY CAROLINE CUNNINGHAM

No part of this book may be reproduced or transmitted in any form or by any means, electronic or mechanical, including photocopying, recording, or by any information storage and retrieval system, without permission in writing from the publisher. For information address: Bantam Books.

Library of Congress Cataloging-in-Publication Data

Pierson, Stephanie.
Vegetables rock! : a complete guide for teenage vegetarians /
Stephanie Pierson.
p. cm.
Includes bibliographical references and index.
ISBN 0-553-37924-0
1. Vegetarianism. 2. Vegetarian cookery. I. Title.
TX392.P53 1999
613.2′62—dc21 98-29570
CIP

Published simultaneously in the United States and Canada

Bantam Books are published by Bantam Books, a divsion of Random House, Inc. Its trademark, consisting of the words "Bantam Books" and the portrayal of a rooster, is Registered in U.S. Patent and Trademark Office and in other countries. Marca Registrada. Bantam Books, 1540 Broadway, New York, New York 10036.

PRINTED IN THE UNITED STATES OF AMERICA

FFG 10 9 8 7 6 5 4 3 2

BUSINESS/SCIENCE/TECHNOLOGY DIVISION
CHICAGO PUBLIC LIBRARY
400 SOUTH STATE STREET
CHICAGO, IL 60605

R01297 34172

Page 99: Recipe courtesy Josefina Howard, Rosa Mexicano, from *Saveur* Magazine.

Pages 113, 117, 146–7: Recipe courtesy *Saveur* Magazine.

Pages 101–2, 166: From *Recipes 1-2-3* by Rozanne Gold, photographs by Tom Eckerle. Copyright © 1996 by Rozanne Gold, text. © 1996 by Tom Eckerle, photographs. Used by permission of Viking Penguin, a division of Penguin Putnam, Inc.

Page 116: From *The Complete Italian Vegetarian Cookbook* by Jack Bishop. Copyright © 1997 by Jack Bishop. Reprinted by permission of Houghton Mifflin Company. All rights reserved.

Pages 133–4, 139, 140–1: From *The Perfect Recipe* by Pam Anderson. Copyright © 1998 by Pam Anderson. Reprinted by permission of Houghton Mifflin Company. All rights reserved.

Pages 134–5, 164–5, 178: From *Feeding the Healthy Vegetarian Family* by Ken Haedrich. Copyright © 1998 by Ken Haedrich. Used by permission of Bantam Books, a division of Random House, Inc.

Pages 143–5: "Golden Tofu, Thai Coconut Marinade, and Caramelized Tofu" from *Vegetarian Cooking for Everyone* by Deborah Madison. Copyright © 1997 by Deborah Madison. Used by permission of Broadway Books, a division of Random House, Inc.

Pages 151–6: Reprinted from *The Classic Pasta Cookbook.* With the permission of Guiliano Hazan and DK Publishing, Inc.

Pages 156–8, 161–2, 167–8: From *Little Meals* by Rozanne Gold. Copyright © 1993, 1999 by Rozanne Gold. By permission of Little, Brown and Company.

Pages 125, 168–9: From *An American Place* by Larry Forgione. Copyright © 1996 by Larry Forgione. Used by permission of William Morrow and Company, Inc.

To Phoebe, the subject of my affections.

To Tom, the object of my affections.

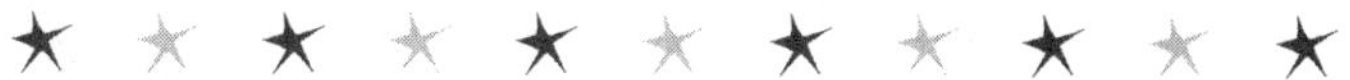

Acknowledgments

To Marcy Posner, Katie Hall, Therese McDonald, Melissa Hamilton, Michelle Daum, Harriet Blumencranz, Heather Willensky, Caroline Schaefer, Christopher Hirsheimer, Dorothy Kalins, Donna Warner, Helene Newman, Alexis Johnson, Megan Connell. For your endless and enthusiastic help/wisdom/insight/encouragement/patience/humor and friendship.

A very special thanks to all the wonderful chefs who contributed to this book: Nadine Ames; Pam Anderson; Peter Berley of Angelica Kitchen in New York, NY; Jack Bishop; Alexis Bondaroff; Louis Centeri of Blanche's Organic Café in New York, NY; Mark Feldman of Mrs. Greens Natural Market in Mt. Kisco, NY; Larry Forgione of An American Place in New York, NY; Christopher Gaddess; Rozanne Gold; John Gottfried of the Gourmet Garage in New York, NY; Ken Haedrich; Melissa Hamilton from *Saveur* Magazine; Giuliano Hazan; John Holm of Sandbox in New York, NY; Josefina Howard; Joan Huey of Blanche's Organic Café in New York, NY; Matthew Kenney of Matthew's in New York, NY; Deborah Madison; Cary Neff of Miraval, Life in Balance Resort in Catalina, AZ; David Page of Home in New York, NY; *Saveur* Magazine; Chris Schlessinger; Brendan Walsh of The Elms Restaurant and Tavern in Ridgefield, CT; Jerry Weinberg of Five Spice Cafe in Burlington, VT; and John Willoughby.

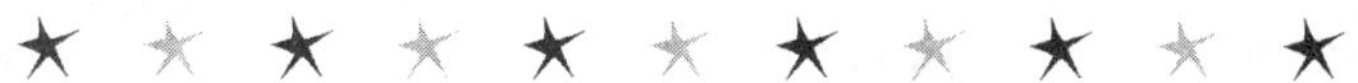

Contents

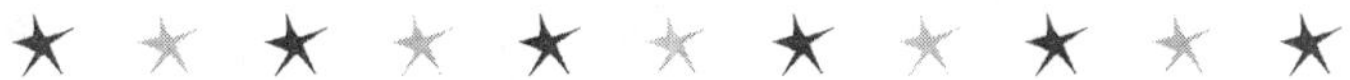

List of Recipes

Great Easy Basics*

Soups, Salads, and Sandwiches

Almost Instant Gratification

All-American Favorites

Un-American Favorites

Pasta

Comfort Food

Sounds Weird but Tastes Great

You Only Live Once: Desserts

* A (v) means the recipe is vegan.

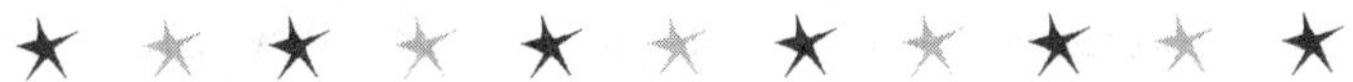

Foreword

"Mom," said my thirteen-year-old daughter, Phoebe, uneasily, "there's something you need to know. Something about me that I hope doesn't upset you." I took an enormous breath and held it. "Mom, I'm a, well . . . a vegetarian." I exhaled.

It could have been worse. It could have been a cult or an enormous Day-Glo tattoo of Kurt Cobain or a pen pal in San Quentin who's getting out soon and wants to come and visit. But take it from me, at the beginning, for parents, teenage vegetarianism is kind of scary. I had so many questions: Does she hate us? Is she getting back at us for something we did? I think she's supposed to eat legumes. What's a legume? I *knew* I should have paid more attention during health class. Do I have to cook tofu? Do I have to *eat* tofu?

But I gave Phoebe a chance. I listened to her newly evolved thoughts on animal rights and reverence for life, and I decided not to serve pot roast for dinner after all.

Parents of new teenage vegetarians need help. More than anything we need to know you won't die from not eating meat. We want to be reassured that you'll grow the way you should, that your bones will be nice and strong, that you'll still have the energy to kick a soccer ball and that you won't be anemic or anorexic. Then, ironically, after you've been a vegetarian for a while, we overreactive parents begin to discover that you are likely to be eating a far healthier diet than most everybody else in America. Not only will you not die, you will be in fabulous shape; you'll feel great; you'll have more energy, lower cholesterol, and lower blood pressure; you'll be getting more fiber and eating less fat, and you'll have far less chance of developing truly awful diseases when you grow up.

If you're a teenager and you've decided to become a vegetarian, there are a few things *you* really need: sympathetic parents, a great hummus recipe, and a couple of smart comebacks for people who can't wait to tell you that being vegetarian is stupid or silly or something you'll outgrow. "Well, if you don't eat meat, what *do* you people eat?" a disgruntled middle-aged woman in California asked her seventeen-year-old vegetarian nephew. "I eat humans," he answered, with a straight face. (Remember the dialogue from *The Addams Family* movie: "Is your lemonade made with real lemons?" And Wednesday's comeback, "Are *your* Girl Scout cookies made with real Girl Scouts?")

Oh, yes, the other thing you could use is a sense of humor. Smile. You're not only the wave of the future, you're one of the biggest trends in America today. There are now more teenage vegetarians in the United States than ever before. While there are no exact numbers, a recent Roper poll showed that 11 percent of girls aged thirteen to seventeen said they don't eat meat at all. A national survey conducted in 1995 showed that 37 percent of all American teens are trying to avoid red meat completely, which is 50 percent more than people a generation older. About 15 percent of the nation's fifteen million college students eat vegetarian during a typical school day.

Why decide to be a vegetarian? While there are many reasons, the main one for most teens is concern for animals. The second biggest reason is caring for the environment. A healthier diet or concern about weight is another reason. (Interestingly, health is the main reason adults give for becoming vegetarian.) Being influenced by friends who are already vegetarian is why some teens decide to reevaluate their thinking and change their diets. And on a slightly less enlightened note, an increasing number of kids are becoming vegetarian because they think it's cool.

Vegetarianism is healthy, it's intelligent, it's enlightened, it's compassionate, it's cool. And best of all, it has the potential to make your parents crazy. Three times a day. Hey, this diet has *everything*. "Let me get this straight," says Christopher Hirsheimer, a food editor and photographer, "my fourteen-year-old who wouldn't even eat whole wheat bread a month ago is now telling me what to buy, cook, eat, and serve? Not to mention accusing me personally of wrecking our ecosystem?"

But whether you're a vegetarian for idealistic reasons or health reasons you (or your parents) probably have a lot of questions. I did. Phoebe did. And I couldn't find a book that answered them. So I wrote one, with her help. I hope it makes it easier for you to achieve your goals.

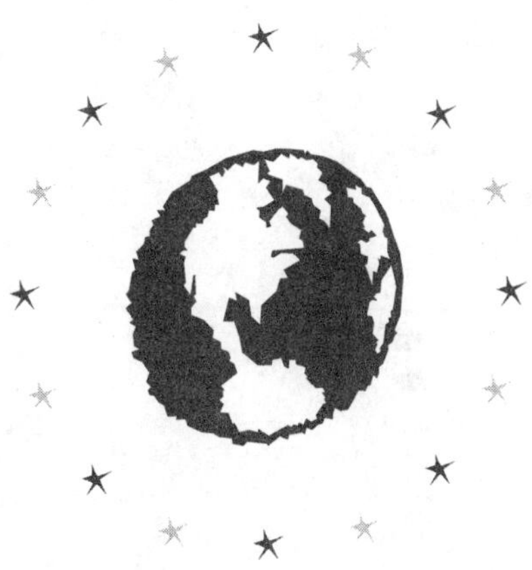

Background

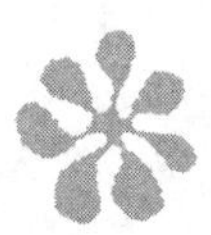

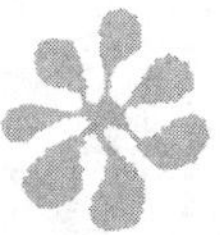

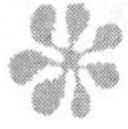

What we eat is within our control, yet the act ties us to the economic, political, and ecological order of the whole planet. Even an apparently small change—consciously choosing a diet that is good for both our bodies and for the earth—can lead to a series of choices that transform our whole lives.

—Frances Moore Lappé, *Diet for a Small Planet*

It can lower your weight, raise your consciousness, save the rain forest, give you energy, save you money, make a cow happy, help your great-grandchildren, challenge the status quo, change the world, and make you fart. Vegetarianism is amazing.

As diets go, vegetarianism is definitely in a class by itself. It has so many distinctions, not least of which is that while it's all about what you eat and what you don't eat, it's not really about food. Philosophically, it's about food as reverence for life. Morally, it's about a compassionate value system. Ethically, it's as much about the health of the planet as it is about our own health. So while vegetarianism is both enriching and nourishing (not to mention satisfying), it is the only diet that can enrich people who aren't even on it.

If you're a vegetarian, you're in good company, from the biggest names in Hollywood to the biggest names in history: Brad Pitt, Drew Barrymore, k.d. lang, Leonardo DiCaprio, Mahatma Gandhi, Leonardo da Vinci, Albert Einstein, Benjamin Franklin, Henry David Thoreau, Charles Darwin, Thomas Alva Edison, and Isaac Bashevis Singer. And don't forget the biggest of them all: the brontosaurus was an early vegetarian.

Even the origin of the word *vegetarian* is worth noting. You might think it has something to do with vegetables. Instead, it comes from the Latin word *vegetare,* meaning "to enliven." Vegetarianism is today what it was fourteen centuries ago—a positive, life-enhancing, enlightened choice.

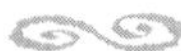

"The greatness of a nation and its moral progress can be judged by the way its animals are reared." —Mahatma Gandhi

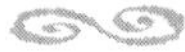

The ideals of vegetarianism originated in ancient Indian literature. Hindus in India have believed for centuries that abstaining from meat will lead to a longer, healthier, more spiritual life. Devotees of yoga believe that foods with a life energy, like vegetables, fruits, and nuts, are necessary to sustain the proper life force. In the fifth century, Buddha popularized vegetarianism. According to the laws of their religion, Buddhists can't slaughter animals, but they can eat an animal as long as they don't kill it themselves.

"But for the sake of some little mouthful of flesh we deprive a soul of the sun and light, and of that proportion of life and time it had been born to enjoy." —Plutarch

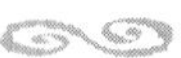

In ancient Greece, vegetarianism was practiced by the Pythagoreans, members of a philosophical and religious sect that existed from the sixth century B.C. to the fourth century A.D. (and who in their spare time devised one of the few math theories I actually understood in school). The Pythagoreans avoided eating any animal, especially fish; they believed it was sinful to harm a fish because fish did not compete with humans for resources.

Other ancient philosophers also came to believe that a diet without meat was simply natural and sensible. Socrates, Plato, Horace, Virgil, and Ovid all shared that point of view.

> *"I have no doubt that it is part of the destiny of the human race in its gradual development to leave off the eating of animals as surely as the savage tribes have left off eating each other when they came into contact with the more civilized."* —Henry David Thoreau

Historically, many cultures have abstained from eating meat. But it wasn't until the middle of the 1800s that Americans became aware of the health and longevity benefits of vegetarianism. In 1843, an experimental vegan community was founded in Harvard, Massachusetts. It was called Fruitlands, and one of its founders was Amos Bronson Alcott, father of the writer Louisa May Alcott. In 1850, the American Vegetarian Society was founded in New York, and the term *vegetarianism* was coined. William Metcalf, a Bible Christian minister in Philadelphia whose sect believed the Bible prohibited meat eating, was largely responsible for these developments.

While the Bible Christians were remarkably enlightened about ethical, environmental, and health issues, they didn't quite get it all right. One of Metcalf's disciples, a minister by the name of Sylvester Graham, preached about the evils of forces he thought too stimulating to be good for us. These included meat, white bread, alcohol, coffee, extramarital sex, and tight pants.

Another enormous religious influence on vegetarianism has been the Seventh-Day Adventist church. For more than 150 years, Seventh-Day Adventists have focused on a healthy diet "for the glory of God." About 50 percent of its church members are vegetarians and close to 100 percent of the clergy. Interestingly, the cancer rate for Seventh-Day Adventists is one-half to two-thirds that of the general population. Hmmm.

The popularity of vegetarianism in America has ebbed and flowed. It flourished from the mid-nineteenth century to the early part of the twentieth century when vegetarian restaurants and retreats opened and vegetarian societies started. The popularity of vegetarianism diminished when the all-American diet of meat and dairy became the standard around the 1950s. In the late 1960s and 1970s, a healthy planetary consciousness and disdain for the establishment (think Woodstock, think *Hair,* think The Grateful Dead) encouraged young people to embrace vegetarianism as part of an alternative lifestyle and to protest the ignorance of anyone unenlightened enough to still eat meat (think parent).

"The fewer animal products you eat, the more earth friendly your diet." —Virginia Messina and Mark Messina, *The Vegetarian Way*

There were two other enormous influences in late twentieth century vegetarianism. One was Frances Moore Lappé's book *Diet for a Small Planet,* written in 1971, which brilliantly laid out for the first time the disastrous effect of food production on our environment and, at the same time, showed that a plant-based diet could easily satisfy all our protein needs. She wrote about the inefficiency of a diet based on animal foods, calling beef cattle "a protein factory in reverse" because cattle actually consume more protein than they provide.

If Animals Are to Talk, We Must Be Their Voices.

—Button worn at a vegetarian rally

The other big influence on modern vegetarianism was the birth of the animal rights movement in the late 1970s and outspoken groups like People for the Ethical Treatment of Animals (PETA), which formed in 1980. These passionate groups made sure, through a combination of advocacy, public relations, and advertising, that the American people were exposed (sometimes in shockingly graphic ways) to the incredibly inhumane methods used in animal agriculture. The combination of growing concern about cruelty to animals and growing environmental issues along with the increasingly clear connection between our diet and our health really hit a nerve.

"Vegetarianism is a kinder, gentler way of looking at the future."

—Harriet Blumencranz, pediatrician

These days it's a pretty simple equation. There's every reason to be a vegetarian. And there's really no reason not to. How can you argue with the facts? Environmentally, pollution and resource depletion from factory farming result in some frightening statistics: In the United States today, half our harvested acreage goes to feed livestock. For example, it takes sixteen pounds of grain and soybeans, not to mention anywhere from twenty-five hundred to five thousand gallons of water to produce just one pound of beef. And did you know five million acres of rain forest are felled every year in South and Central America alone to create pastures for cattle? Here's something else to think about: While grain is fed to animals, hundreds of millions of people in this world go hungry. Finally, this statistic: Production of plant foods is ten to one hundred times more efficient in terms of energy than meat production.

Old MacDonald Had a Farm

The popular image of a farm is that of a peaceful hillside dotted with contented animals—calves frolicking with each other and nuzzling their mothers, or pigs rooting in the earth or rolling happily in barnyard mud, and a group of busy chickens, clucking and scolding and strutting around the barnyard. The reality is that many food animals suffer uncomfortable treatment during their lives.

—Chickens are routinely de-beaked, sometimes at one day of age.
—On egg farms, male chicks have no function and are routinely disposed of.
—Veal calves are likely to spend their entire lives in little crates. They are fed an all-milk diet, which is low in iron and produces anemia, to keep their flesh pale.
—Calves raised for beef are typically de-horned and castrated without anesthesia at a young age.
—On dairy farms, cows are little more than milk-producing machines. Under natural conditions, cows can live for twenty years and will produce milk for ten to twelve years. But today's dairy cows are forced to produce milk in such great amounts that they can do so for only three or four years. Because they are milked by machines and are rarely given a rest from milk production, painful mastitis, or inflammation of the udders, is a common problem for these animals.

—Virginia Messina and Mark Messina, *The Vegetarian Way*

"Nothing will benefit human health and increase the chances for survival of life on Earth as much as the evolution to a vegetarian diet." —Albert Einstein, quoted by John Robbins, *May All Be Fed*

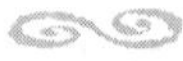

Want to talk about broccoli power? The American Dietetic Association (ADA) says that a vegetarian diet is the most healthful and nutritional way to eat. Population studies have shown that vegetarians tend to have lower rates of obesity, heart disease, hypertension, adult-onset diabetes, and some cancers. The surgeon general has found that nearly 70 percent of all disease is diet related. People eating no meat have 24 percent less heart disease than meat-eaters. People who don't eat meat or dairy have 57 percent less heart disease. Red meat adds more artery-clogging saturated fat to the average American's diet than any other food (*Nutrition Action Newsletter,* June 1997).

Eating Meat Might Be More Expensive Than You Thought

Medical costs, per year, that are directly attributable to America's meat-heavy diet—including the toll taken by high blood pressure, heart disease, cancer, diabetes, gallstones, and obesity—run between $28 and $61 billion, according to Neal Barnard, head of Physicians Committee for Responsible Medicine.

—*Health* magazine, May–June 1996

With data so overwhelming, it's not surprising that vegetarianism is finally in the mainstream in America today. Which doesn't mean that it is necessarily in *your* family's mainstream—a fifteen-year-old from California said, "My mom thinks it's okay and even cooks vegetarian meals for me. My stepdad thinks it is a dumb phase I'm going through—yeah, a three-year phase." Donna Sapolin, editor of *Vegetarian Times,* tells of a young teen who was traveling in the South and was ordering only vegetables from the restaurant menu. "She's a vegetarian," her mother explained to the perplexed waitress. "Oh, I'm so sorry," the waitress exclaimed, looking slightly embarrassed.

If you are a recent convert to vegetarianism, you will discover that there are user-friendly families and user-friendly environments. About half the teens I interviewed or heard from through e-mail had parents who helped them shop for and cook vegetarian food and generally supported them. A fourteen-year-old vegetarian e-mails: "My parents were not and still are not very happy with my choice. They will always support me because this is important to me. They always make a no-meat chili and get lots of pasta and veggies. They deserve an award for raising me."

Pork Queen Squeals

For a while there, everything was going just fine at the annual banquet of the Buena Vista County, Iowa, pork producers. Then the reigning county Pork Queen for the last year, Abigail Boettcher, rose to deliver her farewell speech. A cheerleader, athlete, and daughter of a pig farmer, the college freshman had been a model P.Q. But instead of just thanking the two hundred or so assembled hog pros for a swell year as spokesperson for The Other White Meat, Boettcher decided to announce a bit of personal information: namely, that she's a vegetarian. The news went over like a hog in a hen house. PORK SHOCK, cried one local headline. PORK QUEEN COMES CLEAN read another. "I was nervous about telling them," says Boettcher, "but everybody's been real nice about it."

—*Newsweek*, March 3, 1997

A few had parents who discouraged them, refused to help them, and lectured them about their choice. And while some parents can be difficult, some places can be clueless. C. C. Wagner, a seventeen-year-old vegetarian from South Salem, New York, tells the story of her family's trip to a big-deal New York steak house. It was a celebration and, since C. C. was the only vegetarian, her mother had called ahead to make sure C. C.'s diet could be accommodated. She was assured it wouldn't be a problem. But when they got there, the waiters seemed almost annoyed that C. C. didn't want a steak or lobster. C. C. was horrified when her food was brought to the table: a huge platter overloaded with what looked like vegetarian hospital food: big chunks of plain, watery steamed vegetables, half a head of grayish cauliflower, a whole bunch of carrots, knobby stalks of broccoli, some limp celery stalks. Everyone in the restaurant stared as she sat there humiliated. So while the good news is you may be in the mainstream, the bad news is there will be times you are swimming upstream alone.

There is one animal food that most vegetarians can eat: animal crackers. (Vegans can't eat them because the crackers are made with whey.)

There are types of vegetarians whose diet makes it easier to coexist with nonvegetarians. (These are the vegetarians who actually have a choice at McDonald's and Taco Bell.) And there are really strict vegetarians who need to carefully plan what and where to eat. But basically, no matter what, being a vegetarian means that you don't eat meat, fish, or chicken. Of course, this being a free country, even *that* is open to some interpretation.

The most popular type of vegetarian is *lacto-ovo*. Lacto-ovo vegetarians eat milk, cheese, yogurt, and eggs (animal products). In terms of health, it's generally easy for lacto-ovo vegetarians to meet their nutritional needs. If you eat dairy but not eggs, you're a *lacto* vegetarian. Reversing this, if you eat eggs but no dairy, you're an *ovo* vegetarian.

If you eat no animal products at all—no meat, no fish, no poultry, no dairy, no eggs—you're a *vegan*. Vegan diets are based on vegetables, fruits, grains, legumes, nuts, and seeds. Current figures show that of all vegetarian teenagers, one-third to one-half are vegan. Philosophically, vegans are committed to avoiding animal products and by-products (wool, leather, honey, and cosmetics and soaps derived from animal products), and they abhor any form of cruelty to animals. In addition, vegans believe they have a responsibility to conserve our planet's dwindling food supplies. A newly popular subcategory of vegans are straight-edge vegans, a group committed to caring for the planet and for themselves, who live an alcohol-free and drug-free lifestyle. Straight-edge is an offshoot of the 1980s punk band Minor Threat, whose song "Straight Edge" delivered the message not to drink, smoke, or have sex.

Total vegetarians, or *strict vegetarians,* according to the American Vegan Society, are vegetarians who eat no meat and no dairy but who are committed to vegetarianism more for health reasons than for purely philosophic ones. Either way, both these strict nonmeat, nondairy diets tend to be remarkably healthy—low in fat and high in fiber and protein.

A very different type of vegetarian is called a *fruitarian,* which (no surprise) is someone who eats only fruit (including lots of vegetables that are botanical fruits, like tomatoes, avocados, eggplants, and zucchinis), nuts, seeds, olive oil, and whole grains. It is very difficult to meet all your nutrient needs as a fruitarian so this is not a diet recommended for growing teenagers. Frankly, just the name alone is kind of icky. Imagine you're new at the local high school, you're sitting in the cafeteria, and someone says, "Hey, everybody, meet Harry, he's the new fruitarian in town." There are very few teenage fruitarians in America.

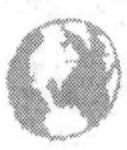

"If your rigid vegan diet is becoming a bore, you might step up to Raw Experience, a 'living foods' restaurant in San Francisco that proudly claims to have staked out the next frontier in meatless cuisine—nothing is cooked here." The Times *goes on to say that Raw's menu transcends mere produce shoveling. It relies heavily on fruit and features items like a fruit-topped pizza. The "crust" of the pizza is created from a mulch of activated buckwheat groats that sits in the sun for half a day. The owner (Juliano, aged twenty-four) says his fruitcentric way of eating makes sense. "Eating fruit and letting the occasional seed pass through our system helps us do our job as fangless, clawless creatures on this planet."*

—*New York Times Sunday Magazine*

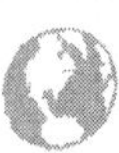

Another vegetarian diet that is as strong philosophically as it is dietetically is *macrobiotics.* Macrobiotics, which is related to Buddhism and, therefore, extremely influenced by Asian philosophy and Asian cuisine, stresses the need for a dynamic and spiritual balance in your life. To achieve this balance, the principles of a macrobiotic diet emphasize eating seasonal foods that are locally produced. Meals are predominantly based on whole grains and sea vegetables (and even occasionally fish). A macrobiotic diet is low in fat and limits the use of foods like nuts and seeds, so this diet can be low in calories as well as low in vitamins and minerals. In general, it is not recommended for teenagers.

Semivegetarianism usually describes someone who doesn't usually eat meat or who doesn't eat certain kinds of meat. There are subtypes of semivegetarians as well: a *pescovegetarian* eats fish and a *pollovegetarian* is a vegetarian who will eat chicken. There's even a group of people labeled *casual vegetarians,* which I thought at first referred to people who wore T-shirts or shoes without socks, but it actually means someone who eats meat only on weekends. Many full-time, fully committed vegetarians (teen and adult) think it makes no sense whatsoever to call yourself a vegetarian and then eat any meat at all. An eighteen-year-old Connecticut college student says, "It makes me a bit crazy when people are wanna-be vegetarians, and I usually tell them so." Sarah, a sixteen-year-old, e-mails her opinion: "If you're going to eat meat, then eat it. None of this 'I'm a preveggie. I only eat chicken.' There's no difference between eating a cow and eating a chicken." A fifteen-year-old vegetarian from New York takes a more resigned view. "Of course, I would rather see the part-time veggies become full-time . . . but I'd rather see people become part-time veggies than not be a veggie at all!"

This part-time vegetarianism, if such a thing isn't a contradiction in terms, is its very own trend. A recent survey showed that fully a third of the twelve to sixteen million Americans who call themselves vegetarian say they still eat chicken or fish. And millions are eating more vegetarian more of the time. According to a

June 1998 Cornell University news release, every year, about one million people adopt a vegetarian diet.

The idea of part-time or occasional vegetarianism does seem to be the answer for enlightened people who know how much healthier vegetables are than meat, but reserve the right to occasionally eat meat. There are an enormous number of cookbooks that now address themselves to these repentant and slightly guilty roast beef eaters. Vegetarians often hear these part-time vegetarians say with a touch of sadness and remorse, "Oh, I wish I could be a vegetarian." As if something were stopping them.

But beyond the existing categories and strict labels of vegetarianism, you can create your own, along with your own reasons. Isabell Moore, a thoughtful nineteen-year-old Columbia University student, feels she isn't always able to be 100 percent committed to the diet she espouses. She calls herself "an aspiring vegan." "I'm trying to be a vegan," she says. "To me it's all about the effort and the trying." Isabell describes her younger sister Margaret as an "involuntary vegetarian" since Margaret is a nonvegetarian living in a very vegetarian household. Anna Thomas, author of the wonderful book *The Vegetarian Epicure,* talks about her own household. "In my world—in my own family, in fact—some are vegetarian and some want to eat meat. Some are even harder to define—the sortavegetarians, I call them."

Full-time, sometime, part-time, occasional, sorta . . . and then there are the vegetarians that make nutritionists blanch and mothers despair. These are the high-fat, low-crunch vegetarians on high school and college campuses all over America who wouldn't be caught dead eating a vegetable. They are the French fry–aterians, pizza-terians, potato chip–aterians, and the fast-food–aterians. Sarah Gray Miller, a New York magazine editor, remembers, "When I was a teenager and I went vegetarian, I spent three months eating Fruit Loops."

Whatever kind of vegetarian you call yourself, there will be a nonvegetarian who can't wait to call you wrong, misguided, deluded, naive, uninformed, crazy. When it comes to food choices (a surprising volatile area) and teenagers (a known volatile area) *everyone* thinks he or she knows what's best for you. Even friends and family and teachers will question your judgment and challenge your beliefs.

Another hard part about being a teenage vegetarian isn't knowing what to eat or not eat, it's knowing what to say or not say. And when not to say it.

How do you know vegetables don't have feelings, too?
So if you don't eat meat, how can you wear leather?
But cows are going to give milk anyway, so why won't you drink it?
No wonder you got strep throat—if you ate meat you'd be a lot healthier.
But if you don't eat meat, what do you eat?

There are a couple of things you can do. One is to form really thoughtful and well-considered responses that actually provide the answers and reasoning behind your choices. And many times this will be enough. But when you're feeling attacked or needled, you're more likely to want to let them have it with a quick, snappy comeback. You obviously have to use your judgment deciding which reply makes more sense. Donna Sapolin, a vegetarian for fifteen years, raises a good point. "If you're a vegetarian because you believe in tolerance and compassion," she says, "why not use that tolerance toward others—be a role model." It's great to have your own cause, but other people have causes, too. So examine your earnestness and have a value system that allows for other points of view.

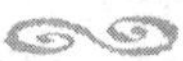

"I didn't fight my way to the top of the food chain to be a vegetarian."

—Anonymous, from the Internet

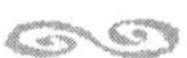

What to Say to a Questioning (Confused/Uninformed/ Doubting) Meat-Eater

—One of my favorite responses comes from a thirteen-year-old vegetarian who has a charming way of mixing her philosophical metaphors. "When people ask me why I'm a vegetarian, I say just put yourself in the animal's shoes and see how you would feel then." (The animal's *leather* shoes?)
—From a seventeen-year-old lacto-ovo: "I just say that I find fried animal muscles nasty."
—From a thirteen-year-old who has been vegetarian for five years: "My choice. Your problem."
—From a sixteen-year-old lacto-ovo: "Well, I can live without the guilt. Can you?"
—From a fifteen-year-old in California: "I'm concerned about the resources wasted on raising animals for food when much of the world's population is hungry and all these people could be fed if we were to switch to a vegetarian diet. So, ultimately, it comes down to the fact that I won't contribute to any system that promotes human suffering."
—From a fourteen-year-old in Iowa: "When someone gives me a hard time, I say 'Pork is for pigs!' "
—From a teenage member of the Vegetarian Society in England: "I quote George Bernard Shaw, who said 'Animals are my friends and I don't eat my friends.' "
—From lots of veg teens: "I won't eat anything with a face."

Nutrition 101

Vegetarian Advice

"124-year-old Jackson Pollard says: 'Avoid alcohol, eat good vegetables, and never, never get married to no skinny woman.'"

—*The Comedian Who Choked to Death*

Lay off the junk food. Eat lots of fruit and vegetables. Eat less fat, use less salt, have less sugar. Don't live on pizza. Eat a varied diet. Spend lots of time at the salad bar and very little time at Burger King. Just say no to Dunkin' Donuts. Take a multivitamin. Stand in the sun for ten minutes every day. Get plenty of exercise and sleep. Don't smoke. Drink your milk, or your soy milk. Give your doctor a call and let him or her know what and how you're doing now that you're not eating meat. Don't forget your protein: eat oatmeal for breakfast and bring a peanut butter sandwich (on whole wheat, not white) to school. Enjoy your food. Think like a squirrel: eat nuts and seeds and grains. Always have the brown rice instead of the white rice. Make friends with soy: tofu, soy milk, veggie burgers. Ask a lot of questions at the health food store. Buy a wok. Laugh a lot. Be nice to your parents.

And that (except for the last two, which I just threw in) is about all you need to know to be a healthy vegetarian.

There is nothing mysterious, complicated, or tricky about being a vegetarian. But you should know what you need nutritionally and the best ways to get it now that you're no longer eating meat. In general, growing teens require more protein, more calcium, and slightly more iron than adults. And special teenagers have their own needs. (Are you playing sports, having your period, pulling all-nighters?) If you are still growing, you need to be aware that your calorie and protein needs will be calculated based on your height, weight, and rate of growth.

You also need to know what to watch out for (like the common tendency for new vegetarians to substitute dairy foods for meat) and what to avoid (Worcestershire sauce, for example, which contains anchovies, which, as you know, are fish and thus a no-no for most vegetarians).

You could probably use a couple refresher courses with titles like Legumes 101, Intro to Vitamins and Minerals, Basic Protein, Beginning Soy. (Could I have slept through *all* of this stuff in college? I guess so. I needed a crash course in *everything*.) You also need to know that different types of vegetarian diets pose different challenges. Lacto-ovo vegetarians, for example, have to worry about whether their diet has too much fat, whereas vegans need to make sure they are getting enough calories and the right vitamins.

"My mother used to make me healthy food when I was a kid. It was so embarrassing." —Deborah Madison, chef, restaurant owner (Greens), and best-selling vegetarian cookbook author

But pay attention in this class; use some common sense, and you'll be just fine. You'll understand nutrition. You'll understand how nutrition affects your diet. You'll understand how your diet affects your body. And you'll know just what to get in the cafeteria at lunch.

You will *not* ever say what I overheard an otherwise bright and well-educated fourteen-year-old say to her friends, in a shocked tone of voice: "Do you know, I just found out there's *fat* in McDonald's French fries?!" Seriously. You will not think that by drinking lots of fruit juice you are getting all the health benefits of fruit (juice lacks fiber, one of the healthier components of fruits and vegetables). You will know that a chocolate-covered granola bar is a high-calorie snack food, not a health food and that many nutritionists think that the new crop of so-called power bars are formulated with lots of hype in every chewy, gooey bite. You'll know that gelatin contains animal by-products.

You won't for a moment think that a free radical is a counterculture revolutionary from Berkeley. (It's a compound that can accelerate the aging process.) And scientists have found that vegetarian diets, which are rich in antioxidants, can fight free radicals and help you stay healthier.

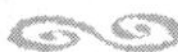

Antioxidant, *by the way, is a hot buzzword in the cosmetic industry, too. You'll see lots of moisturizers and creams that boast antioxidants as part of their formula. The theory is that antioxidants don't have to be in your diet to give you the benefits of younger, healthier-looking skin.*

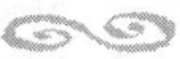

Enough digression. Ready? Let's start with the basics. You need to know about nutrients, vitamins, and minerals. First, what is a nutrient? Nutrients are the substances in foods that help build, maintain, and repair our body tissues. Nutrients fall into six categories: protein, carbohydrates, fat, vitamins, minerals, and water. The nutrients that teenagers have to be most concerned about are protein, calcium, iron, and vitamin B_{12} (Veg Resource Group, *Vegetarian Nutrition for Teenagers*).

Let's start with *protein*. Protein is found in most plant foods. If you eat a varied vegetarian diet and you're getting enough calories, you will be getting all the protein your body needs. Why do you need protein? You can't live without it. Protein is the essential component of every cell in your body. It is required for the synthesis of body tissue as well as for maintaining and repairing existing tissue. In addition, protein maintains supplies of essential enzymes, hormones, and antibodies.

Except for fruit, almost every food of plant origin contains protein—at least a small amount. Some great sources of protein are dairy products, eggs, textured vegetable protein (TVP), soy foods (tofu and tempeh), beans and legumes (they're all beans, but some have a fancy French name just to be confusing), nuts and nut butters (like peanut butter), seeds, and potatoes. (The soybean is an incredible source of high-quality protein. If you're a vegan and not getting any protein from dairy foods, start eating lots of soy.)

At the risk of sounding too technical, protein is made up of amino acids. Eight of these are called "essential" because our bodies can't synthesize them and we can't live without them. Interestingly, no single vegetable food contains amino acids in the proportions that our bodies need. A mixture of proteins is needed to provide the right balance. For example, wheat is low in one amino acid and high in another. Beans are high in one amino acid and low in another. Eat the two foods together and your body's amino acid requirements are met. Most traditional cuisines have recipes that are based on this: rice and beans, pita and chickpeas, rice and tofu.

This kind of combination is called the "complementary protein" theory and was first espoused by Frances Moore Lappé in *Diet for a Small Planet*. Lappé understood that plants could easily meet our protein needs but mistakenly believed that they had to be eaten in certain combinations to be effective. These days, scientists and nutritionists take a much more relaxed approach to all this. The feeling is that if you eat enough protein every day, you will be getting the right amount and the right combinations of amino acids. The proteins you eat at one meal during the day will combine with protein eaten later: your fried rice at lunch is going to rendezvous with your chickpeas at dinner. Your body makes its own complete proteins if a variety of plant foods and enough calories are consumed on a daily basis.

More reassurance: The well-respected *Vegetarian Nutrition Newsletter* says, "Be relaxed about protein. As long as calories are sufficient and the diet is varied, vegetarians easily meet protein needs. It isn't necessary to have a 'high-protein' food like cheese, soy, beans, or meat analogs (tofu dogs or soy burgers) at each meal." How much protein do you need? Well, most Americans on a typical red-meat diet get twice as much protein as they need. Which isn't good. When you consume more protein than you need, it's broken down and stored as body fat, not as a reserve supply to be used later.

Meat Can Kill You

British magazine *Fortean Times* notes the remarkable true story of strict vegetarian Victor Villenti of South Africa who was out jogging when a frozen eight-pound leg of lamb fell from a third-story window and hit him, killing him instantly.

Over the long-term, eating too much protein leads to the risk of heart disease and a loss of calcium as well as the possibility of developing cancer. There are a few food sources with no protein whatsoever: fruits, fats, sugars, and alcohol. So lay off the onion rings in beer batter and the brandied cherries.

Moving right along: *carbohydrates*. There are two types of carbohydrates: simple and complex. Simple carbohydrates are sugars, which can run the gamut from the sugar that is naturally found in fruits and vegetables to the sugar that's unnaturally found in Snickers and Twinkies. Complex carbohydrates are the starchy carbs—pasta and potatoes are what come to mind first. Complex carbs are also found in breads, rice, cereal, vegetables, beans, seeds, and nuts. All carbohydrates, especially complex carbohydrates, give you energy. They're like a high-octane fuel that keeps your body going.

Nutritionist Patricia Johnson, associate dean at Loma Linda University School of Public Health, says that as a rule of thumb, the less meat you eat, the more foods with complex carbohydrates (*not* Snickers and Twinkies) you should add to your diet. She adds that most of these foods also contribute protein to the diet. And rarely does anybody have a bad word to say about complex carbohydrates. They're at the bottom of the Food Pyramid (see page 187), which means they should form the foundation of your diet. Scientists have found that the healthiest populations in the world build their diets around foods that are rich in complex carbohydrates.

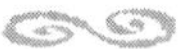

A great bit of nutrition trivia: the more visible seeds a loaf of bread has, the healthier it's likely to be.

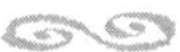

Athletes have always run on them—now it turns out that vegetarians and, in particular, vegans, with their very high carbohydrate intake perform even better than athletes who get some of their carbohydrates from meat (*Veg Way,* 1996). Ounce for ounce, carbohydrates provide the same number of calories as protein and fewer than half the calories of fat.

Now, let's get a little more complex: *Fiber* and *starch* are each a kind of complex carbohydrate, and both have a role to play in a vegetarian diet. Fiber, which is often called "roughage," influences the digestive system. A high-fiber diet helps keep you from getting all sorts of horrible intestinal and bowel diseases that you don't even want to know about. Fiber is found only in plants—no meat contains fiber. The simplest way to get more fiber is to eat more vegetables, fruits, beans, whole grains, and nuts. Bran cereals are great and so is whole wheat bread. Not surprisingly, vegetarians just naturally tend to eat two to four times as much fiber as meat-eaters.

Starch is the main constituent of grains like wheat and barley and oats. Potatoes are also a good source of starch. (Potato chips, alas, don't count since they are just a good source of delicious crunchy fat.) In healthy diets, carbohydrates should provide at least 65 percent of your calories, mostly as starch.

Now on to the American obsession: fat. We love it. We hate it. We can't get enough of it. We get too much of it. Fat is at the tippy-top of the Food Pyramid, with the warning to use sparingly. Your fat requirement is very small. But . . . and this is a big *but* . . . that small amount of fat is absolutely crucial. That's because the only way to get the essential fatty acids your body needs is from fat in your diet. In addition to giving you essential fatty acids, dietary fat transports certain vitamins and prevents deficiencies in those vitamins. Fat's other wonderful talent is to make lots of food taste delicious. The bad news, of course, is that fats are high in calories and too much fat makes us, well . . . fat. The good news is that vegetarian diets tend to be high in fiber and low in fat. Vegan diets are not only low in fat, they're free of cholesterol. (Go, vegans!)

McTrivia

According to the *New England Journal of Medicine*, a whopping 40 to 50 percent of the calories in the average fast-food meal come from fat.

According to *Nutrition Action Newsletter* (July/August 1998), a recent article in *The New York Times* said that three new McDonald's come on line every day, that a corporate goal is to have no American more than four minutes from one of its restaurants. . . .

There are three kinds of fats and one wild card: saturated fat, polyunsaturated fat, and monounsaturated fat along with trans-fatty acid. What's the difference between the fats? Saturated fats are fats that are solid at room temperature. They tend to be found in meats, dairy foods, and some vegetable oils (coconut, palm, palm kernel oil). Polyunsaturated fats are found in vegetable oils, margarine, mayonnaise, and soy foods. They are essential in your diet because your body can't make them. Monounsaturated fat is found in olive oil, canola oil, peanut oil, sunflower oil, avocados, and nuts and is considered the healthiest choice. The fat to particularly watch out for is saturated fat—it should be less than 10 percent of your daily calorie intake. And most doctors think that total fat should be less than 30 percent of your daily calories.

The wild card is the fat that comes from trans-fatty acids. Just the name, *trans-fatty acid,* sounds unappetizing; and sure enough, it's not something you'll want to dig into. Trans-fatty acids are produced when an unsaturated oil, like a vegetable oil, is hydrogenated (hydrogen is added to it), which causes the fat to become solid at room temperature. Because solid fats are less likely to go rancid than liquid fats, food manufacturers hydrogenate the fats in packaged foods, like cookies and cakes, and in margarine to extend their shelf life. Unfortunately, trans-fatty acids may cause heart disease and shorten *your* shelf life, so proceed with caution in the cookie aisle.

No Yolk

Nutritionist Michelle Daum says that egg whites are popular with teenagers in her practice because the whites are high in protein and low in calories (about twenty calories per large egg white). If you cook them at home, Daum says, they're fine. But if you're getting something like an egg-white omelet in a restaurant, watch out for how much fat is being used in the process; it's probably more than you think and more than you want.

POP QUIZ: In the land of fat, which is worse, butter or margarine? Well, the answer keeps changing; but the current thinking is that while butter is bad for your heart, margarine is even worse for your general health because of the trans-fat it contains. Right now, margarine producers are working on reducing the level of trans-fat in soft margarines, so trans-fat-free margarines might be the choice in the future (*Bottom Line/Health*, February 1998). The real answer, of course, is to watch out for both margarine and butter. Also, always try to eat low-fat versions of dairy foods.

Vitamins are essential to your body, although you need them in only very small amounts. Your body can't produce vitamins, so you have to get them through food or supplements. There are thirteen vitamins the human body needs, and vegetarians have to be especially concerned about C, D, and B_{12}. Vitamins are grouped into two categories: water soluble (vitamins B and C) and fat soluble (vitamins A, D, E, and K).

NEWS STORY: Canned Pineapple Runs Rings Around Fresh

According to the *Tufts University Diet and Nutrition Letter*, canned fruits and vegetables usually contain as many or more vitamins as fresh or frozen. That's because produce is canned immediately after it's harvested, preserving nutrients that are lost going from the field to the supermarket. —*Mirabella*, May 1997

Orange juice, grapefruit juice, strawberries, tomatoes, and broccoli are all good sources of *vitamin C*. Getting enough vitamin C by itself is probably not something you have to worry about—vegetarians, particularly vegans, consume a lot more vitamin C than do meat-eaters. But what makes vitamin C particularly noteworthy is that a teenage vegetarian needs to be getting a lot of iron (more about iron later), and one of the easiest ways to increase the amount of iron you absorb from your food is to eat or drink something that's high in vitamin C as part of that meal.

Another important vitamin is *vitamin D.* Vitamin D helps maintain the right levels of calcium and phosphorus in the blood and also helps you absorb calcium, which results in healthy teeth and strong bones. Few foods are naturally high in vitamin D. If you drink milk, you're in luck, because dairy products are fortified with vitamin D. Some brands of soy milk and rice milk are also fortified with vitamin D, as are some breakfast cereals (be sure to check labels). The other way to get it (besides taking a vitamin supplement) is from sunlight—your body can make all the vitamin D you need with enough exposure. If you are out in the sun for ten to fifteen minutes a day, a few days a week during the summer, you'll be fine. Since we can store vitamin D, the amount you make during the summer can last you through the winter when it's much harder for most of us to get enough sun. You know how everybody says always use a sunblock? *Don't* when you're doing your fifteen-minute vitamin D tanning, because even an SPF as low as 8 can block synthesis. Tell your mother when she yells at you (and put on your sunblock after your fifteen minutes of vitatanning).

You pretty much never hear about vitamin B_{12} unless you're a vegetarian, particularly a vegan, and then you never stop hearing about it. The reason is that this vitamin does lots of important things: it helps your body make red blood cells and keeps your nervous system running. If you don't get enough, anemia and irreversible nerve damage can occur. Vitamin B_{12} is readily available in foods of animal origin. So if you're eating meat or dairy products or eggs, you're getting all you need. If you're eating only plant foods, you're not getting any natural vitamin B_{12}. None. Zero.

Hello, vegans. You need to pay special attention to finding foods that are fortified with vitamin B_{12}. Some breakfast cereals (Total and Grape-Nuts, for example), soy milk products, and veggie burgers are good sources. What *aren't* good sources (in spite of manufacturers' claims) are seaweed, tempeh, and miso that *do* have vitamin B_{12} in them but not in a form that our bodies can use. The only plant foods that are reliable sources are fortified. Again, check labels and look for fortified cereals and soy products that you like to eat. And think about taking a multivitamin with vitamin B_{12} just to be on the safe side.

The irony of vitamin B_{12} is that we need so little of it. One teaspoonful is enough to meet the needs of nearly one hundred people for their entire lives. According to the World Health Organization you need only about one microgram of vitamin B_{12} per day. Which is equal to about one-thirty-millionth of an ounce.

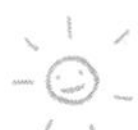

The big question is, How can a vegan diet be considered natural if not one of the foods a vegan can eat includes this essential vitamin? The answer is simple and takes into consideration the evolution of man (not to mention woman). Years and years ago, people got all the vitamin B_{12} they needed from foods that were naturally contaminated with bacteria that synthesize the vitamin. Today, with higher health standards, bacterial contamination is highly unlikely, and fruits and vegetables are no longer a source of vitamin B_{12}.

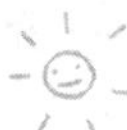

On to minerals. Let's start with *calcium*. Can you say "bone building"? In fact, almost 99 percent of the calcium that's in our bodies is in our bones and teeth. But calcium is not the kind of mineral to rest on this one laurel. It does lots of other terrific things: it helps your blood clot, it helps your muscles contract, it helps your heart beat, and it helps your nerves transmit signals. Most people get their calcium from dairy products. So vegetarians who consume milk, yogurt, and cheese have it relatively easy. Again, it's a little harder for vegans, who need to get their calcium from foods like tahini, tofu (the kind that's processed with calcium sulfate), soy beverages, broccoli, some greens, calcium-fortified orange juice, and cereals.

A short course in how calcium works: We lose calcium every day, through our bodily functions. Our bodies offset this loss by siphoning off calcium from our bones. So the bones in turn lose calcium. This bone calcium *must* be replaced with the calcium we get from the food we eat. So we need a source of calcium every day in our diet to replenish what we're losing.

Our calcium needs change through our lives. Up until the age of thirty, we consume more calcium than we lose. Some experts believe that if you get a calcium-rich diet when you are young, you will lower your risk for soft bones or osteoporosis when you are older.

Something to keep in mind: lacto-ovo vegetarians need to be careful about depending too heavily on dairy foods to meet calcium needs, since the drawback of dairy foods is that they are high in fat, high in calories, and have no iron. A varied diet, with plant foods, fortified soy milk, and calcium-fortified orange juice makes more sense.

Another important mineral is *iron*. Your body needs iron for energy production. If you don't get enough, you'll be very tired and may even be at risk for iron-deficiency anemia. Iron is especially important for teenage girls who are menstruating, since iron is essential for the expansion of blood volume. In fact, menstruating adolescent girls and young women have a high incidence of iron deficiency.

Lots of foods of plant origin contain iron, but this iron is not as easily absorbed as the iron you get from animal sources. So in addition to making sure you get all the iron you need, you have to try to maximize absorption. (If you weren't dozing during the vitamin section, you'll remember that vitamin C helps you absorb iron better, so try to make sure that a meal that includes an iron-rich food also includes a vitamin C–rich food or glass of orange juice.) The reassuring news is that there is no evidence that vegetarian teens are any more or less likely to be iron deficient than teens who eat meat.

Milk: Pros and Cons

You don't need to know this, but it's kind of interesting. We are all raised to think that milk is the perfect natural food and the perfect source of calcium. Milk is sort of all-American and sacrosanct, like baseball and motherhood. Yet it turns out that milk is not essential to our diet. In fact, two-thirds of the world's adult population lack the enzyme to digest milk. All these people consume relatively little dairy food and yet their lower calcium intake doesn't translate into less healthy bones. Even our earliest ancestors got most of their calcium from wild plant foods. Note that there is no other animal on earth that drinks milk from another species. So milk (the good news is it's got calcium, protein, vitamin D, and vitamin B_{12}; the bad news is it's got fat, cholesterol, allergenic proteins, lactose sugar, and often traces of contamination) isn't the only way to get your calcium. Michelle Daum (an adolescent nutritionist in Larchmont, New York, and the author of *Your Overweight Teen: A Handbook*) sings the praises of skim milk, pointing out that it offers outstanding nutritional value: no fat, great protein, great calcium, lots of vitamins, and very few calories. So there is milk and there is milk.

Good plant sources of iron are legumes, iron-fortified cereals and breads, broccoli, spinach, dried apricots, pumpkin and sesame seeds, and something that's always mentioned in iron lists but that doesn't seem like your everyday food: blackstrap molasses. (What *is* blackstrap molasses, I asked Michelle Daum, who wasn't quite sure herself until she looked at the bottle of molasses in her refrigerator and read the label, which confirmed it was just the dark molasses you make gingerbread with. What a perfect excuse to whip up a batch of gingerbread cookies!)

One easy cooking tip is to cook in iron skillets and pots, because research suggests that the iron may pass into the food you're cooking, especially if it's a long-cooking stew. Again, a multivitamin with iron is a good idea.

Zinc is essential for growth, energy production, and repairing body cells. It's really important for teens, because it's particularly crucial to both growth and sexual maturation. As with iron, your body has an easier time absorbing zinc from animal foods than from plant foods. Some good vegetarian sources of zinc are dairy products, legumes, bread, tofu, seeds, nuts, bran flakes, and leafy green vegetables. Interestingly, grains lose zinc when they're processed to make refined flour—which is why it is always a good idea to choose whole wheat or rye over white bread.

To Supplement or Not to Supplement?

Although this country is incredibly into vitamins, most people don't need a supplement at all. The vitamins and minerals already in the food you eat are almost always good enough for you. What you may not know is that lots of the food we eat is already supplemented or fortified. Milk, for example, is fortified with vitamin D; some breakfast cereals have vitamin B_{12}; orange juice is frequently fortified with calcium; and commercial bread has niacin, riboflavin, thiamin, and iron.

There is some question about the worth of supplements in pill form. Too much vitamin E, for example, can interfere with the blood-clotting ability of vitamin K. Too much calcium can inhibit the absorption of iron. Too much folic acid can mask signs of a vitamin B_{12} deficiency. To complicate the matter, there's no absolute level that's known to be just the right amount. Needs vary greatly, based on diet, age, gender, and lifestyle.

What do vitamin and mineral supplements *not* do? They won't correct a diet that isn't healthy to begin with. There's no vitamin you can take to make up for a diet of French fries and pizza. A diet that's too high in calories, fat, or protein and too low in fiber isn't going to change because of a supplement.

What's the answer? Well, after all the enormously sophisticated scientific research, studies, and surveys, the experts' answer is something your grandmother could have told you: eat a balanced diet that's low in fat and high in fruits and vegetables and complex carbohydrates. And as most nutritionists would add, with the special nutritional needs and challenges you face as a vegetarian, taking a daily multivitamin is a simple form of health insurance.

Heads Up! What You Need To Be Concerned About If You Are:

lacto-ovo

Eating all that dairy means it's all too easy to be getting lots of fat (and calories and cholesterol) in your diet from milk and butter and ice cream. Choose the right kind of dairy: skim milk, low-fat cheese, etc. Try to eat a varied diet.

vegan

All the roughage you will be eating can fill you up quickly and the concern is that you won't be getting enough calories or fat. So make sure you don't just bulk up on lettuce and vegetables and fruit. Calcium is another concern since you're not drinking milk (get it instead from calcium-fortified products). Remember that tofu is only a good source of calcium if it has been processed with calcium—check the label. You need to be taking a vitamin B_{12} supplement since almost none of the foods you are eating contain it and only a few are fortified with it. Eat lots of grains, beans (including soy) and you won't have to worry about getting protein.

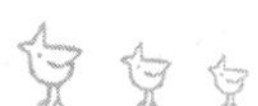

pollovegetarian and pescovegetarian

You don't have to worry about getting protein—just need to make sure you're eating a varied diet with enough fruits and vegetables and complex carbs.

vegetarian and a jock

You need to make sure you're getting enough protein, iron, zinc, and complex carbs for all the calories you'll be burning.

vegetarian and menstruating

You need to make sure you're getting enough iron. Ask your doctor about an iron supplement.

vegetarian and cramming for exams

When you're stressed, you need to make sure you're not living on fast food and junk food. This is a time when your body needs sleep, good food, and nutrients.

vegetarian and dieting

You need to make sure you are getting enough calories and that you're getting them from the right foods. Do not live on Snack-wells and Diet Coke. You also need to make sure that limiting calories (not eating meat and eating fewer calories) isn't the beginning of a body image/eating disorder.

vegetarian and growing

Getting all the necessary nutrients from your diet isn't a problem if you're lacto-ovo. But vegan teens have a harder time (vegan teens actually tend to be shorter than teens who eat animal foods). Vegans who are still growing need to be getting plenty of protein and calories, so emphasis should be on legumes, cereals, nuts/nut butters, and fortified milk substitutes.

teen veg in general

In terms of eating and getting what you need nutritionally, moderation and diversity are a good goal. Also, remember, the less meat you eat, the more complex carbs you should have. Don't obsess about protein. Eat lots of fruits and vegetables. In terms of nutrients, it couldn't hurt to take a multivitamin and if you're vegan, it's pretty much essential. Once in a while (especially at the beginning), go get a check-up from a doctor or have a consultation with a nutritionist. Listen to your body.

some good sources for:	
iron	**calcium**
vegan broccoli potato (with the skin) enriched whole grain bread and cereals dried fruits green beans tomato juice dried beans (all the biggies—kidney, chickpeas, lentils, split peas, etc.) **lacto-ovo** egg yolks plus all the above vegan sources	**vegan** broccoli dark green leafy vegetables (like mustard greens, collard greens, etc.) soy milk (calcium-fortified) orange juice (calcium-fortified) tofu (processed with calcium sulfate) **lacto-ovo** milk (whole, low-fat, skim) cheese yogurt plus all the above vegan sources
vitamin a	**vitamin c**
vegan apricots (dried) asparagus broccoli cantaloupe carrots green peppers peaches plums tomatoes (and lots more fruits and vegetables) **lacto-ovo** fortified milk products egg yolks plus all the above vegan sources	**vegan** citrus fruits: oranges (orange juice), grapefruit (grapefruit juice), tangerines, lemons broccoli cantaloupe potatoes strawberries tomatoes (tomato juice) (and more fruits and vegetables) **lacto-ovo** exactly the same as the above vegan sources

<table>
<tr><th colspan="2">some good sources for:</th></tr>
<tr><th>vitamin b_{12}</th><th>vitamin d</th></tr>
<tr><td>vegan
no sources of b_{12} in the vegan diet

lacto-ovo
milk
yogurt
eggs
cheese</td><td>vegan
look for foods like cereals fortified with vitamin d or consider supplements or use sunlight as a source

lacto-ovo
fortified milk is the only reliable dietary source
plus all the above vegan sources</td></tr>
<tr><th>zinc</th><th>protein</th></tr>
<tr><td>vegan
whole grain breads and cereals

lacto-ovo
milk
egg yolks
plus all the above vegan sources

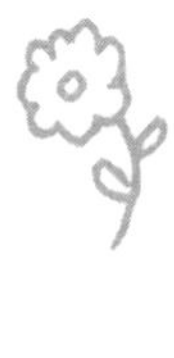
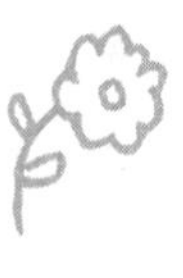
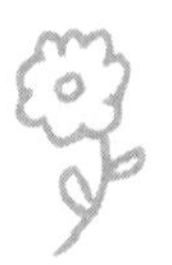</td><td>vegan
all soy products
nuts and seeds
beans and legumes (this includes peanuts and peanut butter)
grains (this includes cereal, pasta, bread, rice, potatoes)

lacto-ovo
eggs and dairy (yogurt, all kinds of milk and cheese, except for cream cheese which is not a source of protein)
plus all the above vegan sources

NOTE: You do get some protein from vegetables, just not enough to put it on the list. For best nutrition, remember to eat a variety of protein-rich foods.</td></tr>
</table>

chapter 3

★ ★ ★ ★ ★

Fast Food. Junk Food. Health Food. Good Food. Vegetarian Food. Help!

You've decided to be a vegetarian, and it's amazingly easy. At school, there's a huge and ever-changing assortment of salads, soups, grilled vegetables, tortillas, curries, and even a selection of fruit smoothies and fresh-squeezed juices. Your fellow students applaud your efforts to avoid meat and do what they can to help. Not once do they "Moo!" or "Oink!" at you when they eat meat.

At home, your supportive family is happy to help you make home-cooked vegetarian stews and casseroles as well as tasty, nutritious snacks. They even joined an organic food co-op to make it easier for you. Thanksgiving? No problem—your loving grandmother made extra side dishes for you and never once insisted you try just one bite of turkey.

Your town is great—there's a wonderful Indian restaurant with vegetable curries and fresh, fragrant potato breads. There's a Japanese restaurant with a delicious miso soup and a sushi bar for veggie cucumber or oshinko (pickled vegetable) rolls. The local Italian trattoria has homemade pastas and fresh tomato sauces. Of course there are a couple of local Moosewood-type restaurants where you always feel comfortable. The health food store in town is big, friendly, inexpensive, and delivers. Free of charge. Your supermarket is the best—tons of fresh organic and ethnic foods, a whole frozen vegetarian section, so many brands of granola and soy milk and veggie burgers that there's always something new to try.

Even the local fast-food restaurants have delicious nonmeat options, and the well-informed people who work there know everything about the ingredients and food preparation so you can always be sure of what you're getting. There are two farmers' markets within walking distance of your house. No . . . they're right in front of your house. Plus, you've got your own incredible garden with ripe tomatoes and sweet melons and even tropical fruits, like golden pineapples and juicy papayas. . . .

Okay, it's a fantasy. And the reality is that the salad bar at your school is pathetic—their idea of salad fixings is iceberg lettuce, three-bean salad from a jar, and that bottled ranch dressing that's the same shade as Pepto-Bismol. Your town doesn't have a health food store. But it's got two steak houses and a rib joint. The organic bananas in your supermarket cost twice as much as regular bananas, *and* they're brown and spotted.

At Thanksgiving, your grandmother says she can't believe that *this* is when you choose to make some sort of statement, and she hopes you're happy ruining the holiday for everyone else in your family. Your mom gets home from work at 7:00 and isn't in the mood to cook one dinner, let alone two. Your dad (only visiting this planet) can't remember which part of the spaghetti and meatballs it is that you can't eat. You have four hours of homework and no time to cook, so you microwave some leftover pizza and round out the meal with half a bag of Doritos and a Coke. Do you think Gandhi ever had to pick Bac*Os out of a salad to make it vegetarian or explain to the guy at McDonald's that he would like the cheeseburger with everything except the burger?

Meet the Mirbachs!

The Mirbachs live in New Canaan, Connecticut. Mrs. Mirbach eats meat. Mr. Mirbach is a vegan. Their thirteen-year-old son is crazy about McDonald's and hot dogs. Their fifteen-year-old daughter is a lacto-ovo vegetarian. "How many meals do you cook every night?" I ask Cynthia Mirbach, in an awed tone of voice. "Oh, I've stopped cooking," she replies.

She's kidding. At least, I think she's kidding.

What's striking about the new all-American family is that it isn't all anything at all. This family is meat-eating, strictly vegan, pure lacto-ovo, and crazy about fast food. What makes it work for the Mirbachs? "Everyone accepts everyone's eating habits," says Cynthia Mirbach. "So I guess the answer is tolerance, plus lots of pasta and salad."

There may be twelve to sixteen million Americans who call themselves vegetarian, but why does it sometimes seem like half of them live in Berkeley and the other half live in New York City and you live in, say, Indiana or Texas or New Hampshire? "I love my adoptive state," says vegetarian cookbook author and chef Ken Haedrich who lives in Rumney, New Hampshire. "But I have to admit—somewhat sadly—that our restaurant scene is not exactly on the cutting edge of innovative vegetarian cooking. In fact, the one totally vegetarian restaurant in the state just went out of business."

A diet rich in fruits and vegetables roughly halves overall cancer risk.

—Quoted by *Glamour,* June 1997

And that's exactly the state vegetarianism is in. In many ways, there's never been a better time to be a vegetarian. It's definitely the wave of the future; but unfortunately, the present hasn't quite caught up. "I'd love a cookbook," a fifteen-year-old vegetarian says, "with recipes where I don't have to go to India to get the food." "If they ran out of milk at school, it would be a big crisis," says a Florida college freshman. "But when there's no more soy milk, it can take weeks for them to order more." "You couldn't be vegan and go to my school, Western Carolina University," states a student there, "unless you wanted to eat salad all day."

In a world that is supposedly more health conscious and environmentally aware than ever, what does it say about us that the number one, two, and three growth items in restaurants in recent years have been hamburgers, hot dogs, and sodas? Or that the percentage of people now suffering from obesity is at a record high? Or that fewer than one-third of adults in America participate in any regular physical activity? Or that in a national survey, over a three-day period, about 30 percent of teens did not eat any fruit at all?

Welcome to the real world. Where the arches are golden, the saturated fat is sizzling, and most people still think that if you're vegetarian it's okay for you to eat fish.

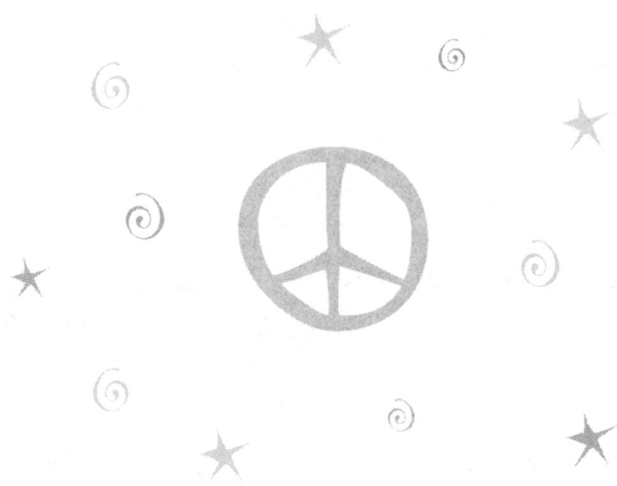

A conversation I wrote down, verbatim, between Phoebe (who had only been vegan for a few months) and the (highly intelligent) wife of our dry cleaner. To protect her, we'll refer to her as "Mrs. Martinize."

MRS. MARTINIZE TO PHOEBE: How's your vegetarianism going?
PHOEBE: Great, thanks.
MRS. MARTINIZE: What is it you don't eat?
PHOEBE: Meat, dairy, meat by-products.
MRS. MARTINIZE: Now, do you eat any fish?
PHOEBE: No, vegetarians don't eat fish.
MRS. MARTINIZE: Oh, I didn't know that. You know what always struck me as odd?
PHOEBE: No, what?
MRS. MARTINIZE: Well, the people in health food stores. They're all skinny and pale. And they sort of seem like zombies. Do you know what I mean?
PHOEBE: Well, not . . .
MRS. MARTINIZE: (interrupting her) You don't look that bad yet. (pauses) Of course, you haven't been vegetarian that long.

To be a successful vegetarian in this somewhat schizophrenic world, you're going to have to wrestle with a couple of inconsistencies and puzzles. One: if it's clear beyond a shadow of a doubt how much healthier you'll be if you eat lots of fruits and vegetables and pretty much stay away from meat, how come so many people still choose to eat meat? How come there are approximately six thousand steak houses in America today? And what's with the poll commissioned by the National Cancer Institute in 1991 that showed only 8 percent of Americans thought vegetables were important? (Once you figure that out, maybe you can figure out why my husband still smokes.)

Two: if you've decided not to eat meat and you don't want to compensate by eating lots of junk food, how come everyone seems to make it so hard to do this? Ever try to find hummus or tabouli or whole wheat pita or a really fresh fruit salad at the neighborhood deli? Ever go to a Major League Baseball or National Basketball Association game and ask the guy selling red hots if he has tofu dogs instead? Ever try to find anything nonfried, let alone nonmeat at the food court in a mall?

And one more thing: if foods that are filled with fat are so bad for you, how come they taste so good? "I jog, I watch what I eat, I meditate," says a California dietician. "And when I go to the movies I always get a big tub of popcorn, the kind that was popped in that awful coconut oil and I eat the whole thing." A nutritionist told me about the time Dr. Nathan Pritikin, the guru of low-fat, went to a university nutrition conference and proudly offered everyone his newest find: a nonchocolate, nonfat, nondairy chocolate cake that had fewer calories than a small grapefruit. While everyone else politely nibbled this tasteless wonder, one lone dietician politely declined. When asked why, she explained that she would rather have one gorgeous, rich, gooey, incredibly decadent piece of real chocolate cake once a year than have to settle for a perfectly engineered, perfectly awful mutation you could eat all the time. Even the dieticians can't stay on their diets!

To make it all work, you need to be realistic, you need to be flexible, you need to be creative, you need to be tolerant, you need to be well-informed, you need to read labels, and you need to believe that *you can survive* in vegetarian-challenged places like ballparks, rib joints, airplanes, fast-food courts, and school cafeterias, even in New Hampshire.

Dilemma of a Hungry, Health-Conscious Vegan

"I can't eat the cookies I like, even though they're all natural because 'natural' means they have eggs and milk and butter in them. But, as a vegan, I can eat the cookies made with chemicals and additives and preservatives and artificial ingredients and fake colorings. What's wrong with this picture?" —Phoebe Connell

Some survival tips. First, school cafeterias. The good news is that junior high schools, high schools, and colleges are trying harder than ever. They know there's a lot of you, and they are offering vegetarian options. Colleges are better than high schools. Nine out of ten offer a complete vegetarian menu; and many offer vegan alternatives, sometimes with interesting results. According to Karen Dougherty, executive dietician at Yale, "We have definitely noticed students are eating down the food chain—meat-eaters eat vegetarian a couple of times per week and vegetarians regularly eat the vegan option." Colleen Reid, at Brown University, offers one reason why. "I've found that many people who would normally eat meat, don't at college, because dining hall food is just not very good, especially the meat. This causes some people to become vegetarians and others to only eat meat at home or when going out to dinner."

Some Tips for Making It Easier

—A seventeen-year-old vegan who occasionally misses meat and who is not all that crazy about vegetables, likes to sprinkle A.1. sauce on his steamed broccoli, carrots, etc.
—To make grapefruit taste a little sweeter, vegetarian chef Ken Haedrich spreads raspberry preserves on a grapefruit half.
—Make one monthly trip to a food co-op or health food store and stock up. Mail-order stuff.
—If the vegetarian entrée in your college cafeteria is unacceptable, make nachos. Just put cheese on chips, microwave, and add salsa (from Saisha Uma-Michelle Grayson).
—In a pinch? Get plain rice in the cafeteria and sprinkle on tamari sauce (from Saisha Uma-Michelle Grayson).
—Freeze green grapes. They taste sweet and icy.
—Peanut butter turns an apple or banana from a boring fruit to a surprisingly delicious snack.
—Puree cottage cheese in a food processor. Add some herbs, then use as a spread on toasted bagels.

The bad news for many younger vegetarian teens, who have no time to eat and zero interest in following the Food Pyramid ("let's see . . . let me get my two daily servings of legumes . . ."), vegetarian food is most likely to be a bagel or French fries or slice of pizza. By college, the food is likely to be better, and their diet is likely to be, also. According to a survey done by the *Vegetarian Journal*, many schools are actively looking to add more nonmeat options. Some universities are on the verge of creating vegetarian dining halls. And in some remarkably enlightened colleges, more than half the student body is vegetarian, which makes for some great vegetarian food and some unusual complaints. "The only prejudice I've found," writes a Sarah Lawrence freshman where half the student body is vegetarian, "comes from the carnivores who feel we've dominated food services. For example, our school serves very little red meat and will have meals once in a while with no meat options." A sophomore at an Ivy League college says, "It's actually easier to be a vegetarian at school than at home. Here there's always tofu and beans and rice and baked potatoes and salads."

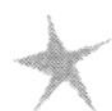

Most Popular Dishes in College Cafeterias

1. Pasta with meatless sauces
2. Vegetarian lasagna
3. Pizza
4. Mexican specialties
5. Vegetable stir-fries

—From a National Restaurant Association survey

Some schools get rave reviews. "Some of the best vegetarian food I've ever had was at college," says a Tufts University alumna, who explains that because of the enormous influence of the health and nutrition center at Tufts, an inordinate amount of energy and resources have been spent on creating healthy and delicious meals for undergraduate and graduate students. And some schools make you work a little harder. A vegan freshman at Columbia University says that putting together a good lunch in the cafeteria is like everything else at a large university—you have to learn the drill. "After a few months," she says, "I learned you get vegetables from the grill, go over to the salad bar and get the rice, go back to the vegetarian table and add the tofu, then take it all back to the grill guys and ask them to sauté it."

Of course, one of the best ways to find out whether a college is sympathetic to a vegetarian lifestyle and dedicated to presenting an appealing vegetarian cuisine is word of mouth. Ask your friends who go there. And don't expect that because a college is in a health-conscious kind of town that it will be an ideal choice for vegetarians. "Boulder is a really cool place," says a University of Colorado senior, "but I found that the food in the cafeteria was surprisingly boring—not much variety . . . very few fresh vegetables." And for all of a college's good intentions, don't expect miracles. "As always," e-mails a freshman at a small liberal arts college, "finding decent vegetarian food is a challenge. In fairness, making good food for large amounts of people in a cafeteria style is not easy; and from what I can tell, the quality of all food choices, meat or nonmeat, seems to be pretty consistent in its general mediocrity."

Maybe the only thing harder than making good food for large amounts of people is making it fast. Getting healthy and nutritious food (vegetarian or not) in fast-food restaurants is hard. And most people don't go to fast-food places when they want a healthy, well-rounded meal. But in general, keep in mind that a ridiculously high percentage of the calories in a fast-food meal comes from fat, and try to choose sensibly. You're probably better off at places that serve burritos instead of burgers. Wherever you go, choose something that's broiled or grilled, not fried. At the salad bar, stay away from the macaroni salad, potato salad, and fattening dressings. Skip the (meaty, fatty, artificially made) gravy. Have skim milk or fruit juice or a fruit smoothie instead of a milk shake. At breakfast, skip the cheese and egg croissants and settle for poached or scrambled eggs or have pancakes or French toast without the butter and syrup.

Things to Worry About When You're Eating Out

1. What did they cook the French fries in?
2. The vegetables were grilled on the same grill as the meat.
3. There is MSG in the stir-fried vegetables.
4. The vegetable soup was made with chicken broth.
5. The knife that cut the meat cut the vegetables.
6. There's cheese in the burritos.
7. There's lard in the pie crust.
8. There's egg in your vegetable dumplings.
9. Your vegetable fried rice or lo mein is made with an egg.
10. There's butter and cream in your pasta primavera.
11. The rice was made with butter.
12. There's milk, eggs, and/or butter in the bread.
13. The salad croutons were fried in lard or made with egg.
14. The refried beans were made with lard.

Some good choices at fast-food places are garden salads, vegetarian pizzas (cheeseless for vegans), bean burritos, baked potatoes (top with vegetables and skip the sour cream), an assortment of vegetable side dishes, and veggie burgers or heroes. *Vegetarian Journal*, published by the Vegetarian Resource Group (VRG), surveyed over one hundred fast-food and casual restaurant chains (what they serve, fat content, hidden nonvegetarian ingredients, etc.), and they periodically update their findings. If you send $3.00 to VRG, P.O. Box 1463, Baltimore, MD 21203, they'll send you the latest information. Some of the findings are encouraging: almost all the restaurant chains surveyed now use all-vegetable shortening for frying. VRG points out that even fast-food chicken places now offer vegetarian offerings: a vegetarian can go to KFC and lunch on an ear of corn, mashed potatoes, and cole slaw. At Boston Market and Kenny Rogers Roasters, you can get a choice of three side orders on a sampler plate. Subway is now offering the most enlightened array of nonmeat, low-fat subs.

Oh My God, I Ate a Chicken McNugget!

PART 1: "Listen to your body. Your needs have a lot to do with your growth. If you ever do eat meat, you shouldn't feel guilty about it. It's just like dieting. You need to realize you haven't violated anything."

—Dr. Harriet Blumencranz

PART 2: "After you lapse you feel bad. You know you're kind of mad. Then you take it all a little easier. Because it's really all about reverence for food. Maybe it sounds a little New Age, but vegetarianism is about putting things in your body you should feel proud of."

—Isabell Moore, Columbia University

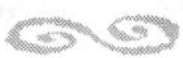

Is it vegetarian or *vegan?* If you're not sure about something that's served in a restaurant, ask. If the employees aren't sure, don't order it. And you can't tell by looking. The flour tortillas at Wendy's contain whey, so they're not vegan; but Wendy's taco chips, taco sauce, and taco shells *are* vegan. The Italian dressing at Pizza Hut is vegan but contains MSG. Some pizza crusts contain dairy products. Some guacamole is made with mayonnaise. Ask.

If fast-food places are a little challenging, dining out in regular restaurants can be vegetarian heaven. Especially ethnic restaurants. *Especially* ethnic restaurants where the emphasis is so skewed toward grains and vegetables that your choice is huge. Japanese, Tibetan, Thai, Vietnamese, Egyptian, Indian, fusion cuisines, macrobiotic—there's a world of amazing tastes and flavors out there. You might not like everything, but chances are you will be rewarded for your willingness to try new foods. The Japanese know how to make incredible tofu dishes. They should—they've been doing it for centuries. Vegetables aren't something you *have* to eat in Italy; they are the stars of a dazzling pasta primavera or rich minestrone soup. And at the risk of sounding corny, a country's cuisine can be an introduction to that country's entire culture.

What else is great? Crunchy Chinese stir-fries, vegetable fried rice, tangy hot-and-sour soups, vegetable tempuras, cucumber sushi rolls, Japanese soba noodles simmered in vegetable broth, vegetable curries served with cool mango chutney and potato bread, freshly stuffed grape leaves, vegetable paellas, creamy Italian risottos flavored with wild mushrooms, golden polenta cakes, Spanish onion and potato frittatas, Moroccan green sauce, Vietnamese spring rolls with peanut dipping sauce, sesame noodles with spring asparagus. I have to stop. I'm getting hungry.

And if you're lucky, there are American restaurants and cafés near you where tofu and fresh broccoli rabe and chickpea beans are not considered foreign foods but are part of the growing American vegetarian cuisine. There are the meccas like Moosewood in Ithaca, New York; Blind Faith in Evanston, Illinois; Angelica Kitchen and Souen and Zen Palate and Blanche's Organic in New York; and Greens and Millennium in San Francisco. And there are thousands of other places from Florida to Oregon where people really care about wholesome, delicious, natural foods. Where it's all about fresh herbs and seasonal produce, wonderfully savory stews served with loaves of sourdough bread still warm from the oven. Where dishes as basic and homey as vegetarian chili, black bean soup, macaroni and cheese, vegetable lasagna, fried green tomatoes, and bread puddings are perennial favorites.

And you'll be happy to know that this is one area where you're In with the In Crowd: a recent poll commissioned by the National Restaurant Association showed that one in five diners say they now go out of their way to choose restaurants that serve at least a few meatless entrées (*Health* magazine, May–June 1996). Again, most of the same fast-food rules apply: stay away from really fattening foods, remember that deep-frying is the enemy of the people, ask if you're not sure about an ingredient or an additive, and go for grains and beans and greens. And I would suggest (I *am* a mother) that you try new cuisines and new foods as often as you can. Be open-minded.

The Vegetarian Resource Group, with the help of its readers, has put together the Vegetarian Journal's Guide to Natural Foods Restaurants. *There are listings for more than two thousand restaurants, juice bars, delicatessens, and travel spots. It's available for $14.00 (including postage) from VRG, P.O. Box 1463, Baltimore, MD 21203 (Phone: 410–366–VEGE). Overseas, there's the* European Vegetarian Guide: Restaurants and Hotels, *which is also available through VRG. It's $16.00 (including postage). Online, the "World Guide to Vegetarianism" Web site (www.veg.org/veg/Guide) lists restaurants by country, state, city, and vegetarian category. Call ahead, though, if you can, since restaurant information (like food) can go stale quickly.*

Ken Haedrich (the man who manages to remain a happy vegetarian in New Hampshire), describes in his book *Feeding the Healthy Vegetarian Family* what it's like to eat out in some less sympathetic restaurants. The kind where the waitress insists on telling you about the surf-and-turf special, even though you've already asked for the vegetarian offerings, and who thinks that if you don't eat meat or fish perhaps you would like the coq au vin because the chicken is free range.

Yes, luncheonettes, diners, old established neighborhood restaurants, and cafés can be completely clueless. Somehow they've been serving the same menu with the same dishes forever, and the possibility of them putting a veggie burger on the menu is about as likely as them taking away that little bowl of pastel mints next to the cash register. We go to a local diner that has *everything* (371 items on the menu), *including* revolving desserts and those pastel mints. And yet there are only 18 dishes that a vegan can eat. How to make it all easier for everyone? Ken Haedrich has a few rules that make a lot of sense.

rule #1: When you speak to restaurant people, be explicit about your dietary guidelines. Don't say: *I'm a vegetarian.* Say: *I'm a vegetarian. I don't eat meat or seafood but I do eat eggs and dairy products.* Or *I don't eat meat or fish, but I will eat just about anything else except the stuff the fellow at the next table just sent back.* Get it? This initial introduction will help narrow down the field and quickly clue in your waitress to your preferences so she can help you out.

rule #2: Always call ahead before trying a new restaurant. Or at least try to. You can tell a lot about a restaurant's receptivity to vegetarians by the way they handle you on the phone. Call between meals and ask to speak to the chef or kitchen manager. [MY NOTE: Or make your parents do this and tell them you have a lot of homework.] He or she should be willing and able to talk to you intelligently about the sort of food you would like. And you should get the distinct impression that the chef knows something about meatless cuisine and looks to feeding you as a creative challenge, not as a pain in the patootie. If the chef mumbles something about a baked potato and the salad bar, this is not a good sign. It is clearly in the chef's best interest to accommodate you, and if he or she can't figure that out, don't bother. Our favorite restaurant is Italian, not vegetarian, but the chef literally knocks himself out for us whenever we go there; consequently we go there very often.

finally, rule #3: If you do get a good meatless meal, let the chef know. Chefs are not known for their small egos; and the more you can express your gratitude for a job well done, the better the kitchen is going to take care of you. Tell the waitress and chef you appreciate their efforts. If you do, tell them you feel strongly about supporting places that cater to vegetarians; then tell your friends. Don't be afraid to drop specific hints about the sort of vegetarian foods you like and would *love to try* if the chef ever made anything like that. Most good chefs like a challenge, and they'll do everything they can to keep you happy.

Up in the air about what to eat? Call ahead to order a vegetarian meal or fruit plate on a plane (ask your travel agent to call or just call the airline reservation number yourself). Beware the hidden ingredient in these meals: fat. A couple of years ago the Physicians Committee for Responsible Medicine did a survey of so-called low-fat meals that different airlines offer. (Is there anything in America that hasn't been surveyed at least once?) They found that the meals differed in fat as much as 41 percent.

1. United Airlines: Vegetarian steak and pasta with curry sauce. Percentage of fat: 6.3 percent.
2. Continental Airlines: Green pepper stuffed with spicy vegetarian chili, nuts, and raisins. Percentage of fat: 27.7 percent.
3. TWA: Lentil stew with biryani rice. Percentage of fat: 28.4 percent.
4. American Airlines: Jasmine rice with vegetables and red pepper coulis. Percentage of fat: 28.8 percent.
5. Northwest Airlines: Grilled polenta. Percentage of fat: 32.7 percent.
6. Delta Airlines: Vegetarian spinach ragout. Percentage of fat: 47.9 percent.

Meanwhile, back on earth. A few random thoughts on living in a less-than-perfect world. Do *not* be an evangelical vegetarian. You know the kind: "You're going to eat that piece of chicken? Do you know how that chicken lived? How it died?!" *[Make face.]* It doesn't help. That kind of completely emotional attack only obscures any really rational and thoughtful conversation you might initiate instead (after everyone's eaten). And don't get caught up in My Vegetarianism Is Better Than Yours. It's not a competition. Nor is it a status symbol. Someone who has cut out all meat and all dairy is not on a higher moral plane than someone who's just cut out meat. There are no better or worse vegetarians.

Be an activist. I'm not talking about doing community service or supporting, say, an animal rights organization, although that is great. I'm talking about writing letters to companies and stores and expressing your feelings. You can't believe how effective it can be. And how good you'll feel. Tell a cosmetic company you think it's wrong that they test on animals. Tell a food manufacturer that you can't understand why they can't make their pizza crust without whey. Tell the parent company of the fast-food place that its salad bar never seems very fresh. Tell the health food store that their prices are too high. First of all, you're helping your fellow vegetarians. Second, people in charge can be much more responsive and caring than you think. Make the effort. Chances are they'll respond.

Finally, there *is* a way to guarantee you'll eat great food—just what you're in the mood for, just the way you like it—in a place where you'll always feel right at home. At home. Learn to cook, and a whole new delicious vegetarian world is yours.

Everybody Doesn't Like Something

Do you remember the old Sara Lee slogan? "Everybody doesn't like something. But nobody doesn't like Sara Lee." Clever, charming, a wonderfully positive use of negatives. What made me think of it recently was feeding my beloved nuclear family who, in their eating habits, perfectly illustrate the first half of the slogan, "Everybody doesn't like something," and stop right there.

The specific meal that made me really think of the Sara Lee slogan was a dinner I was attempting to make to please each and every picky palate. I found a recipe in a food magazine for black bean and vegetable burritos. It seemed okay. Simple, healthy, meatless for my teenage vegan. Hearty, filling, kind of familiar for my husband. Low-calorie, flavorful, slightly exotic for me. "It's got grilled vegetables in it? I *hate* grilled vegetables," said Phoebe when she saw me chopping. "I can do it with roasted vegetables if you want," I told her. "Roasted vegetables? I don't like *any* of those vegetables," Phoebe decided. "What's that?" asked my husband. "Cilantro," I replied. "You know cilantro makes me sick," he said. "Can't you make it without cilantro?" Phoebe couldn't eat it with the suggested toppings: shredded Cheddar and sour cream (dairy). Tom couldn't eat it with the chopped tomato (too acid for his stomach). Phoebe didn't want the chile peppers because it would be too spicy.

Among our tastes, our diets, and our philosophies, one of us or some of us or all of us is presently eating no meat, no cheese, no milk, no eggs, no butter, no margarine, no fish, no grilled vegetables, no weird vegetables like fennel or okra, no take-out Chinese, no sushi, no pizza, no fried foods, no fast foods, no artificially sweetened foods, no exotic herbs, no overtly healthy health foods.

So I guess I'm cooking up a new slogan: Everybody doesn't like everything and nobody doesn't like nothing.

chapter 4

★ ★ ★ ★ ★

What to, How to, Ingredients, Techniques, Moral Support

I think one of the benefits of being a vegetarian is that you learn more about food, because you have to make more of an effort.

—Matthew Kenney, owner of the New York Mediterranean restaurants Matthew's, Monzu, and Mezze

The only problem with being a vegetarian is that you have to eat vegetables. Now, if you grew up like I did in the 1950s, that meant you believed most vegetables came from a can, and what didn't come from a can you could get frozen in blocks from the supermarket. At my house, the canned green beans, all limp and waterlogged, were boiled to a fare-thee-well (even though they were already cooked) before they were considered ready to be served. The boxes of frozen lima beans and peas and spinach never quite escaped that cryogenic state once they were defrosted and (sort of) brought back to life. Except for corn (fresh for a few weeks in the summer, otherwise canned and creamed), succotash (frozen), mixed vegetables (canned or frozen), tomatoes (fresh in the summer, otherwise canned), and carrots (fresh but must have been fresher when they were shipped from California two months earlier), there weren't any other vegetables in the world.

To the best of my memory, boiling was the cooking method of choice. Seasoning consisted of adding salt and a lump of butter to the serving bowl. I think back and wonder, Were the vegetables being punished for some reason? Were my brother and I being punished? What had an innocent string bean or tender sweet pea ever done to deserve such a cruel fate?

Today, vegetables are highly evolved and ridiculously likable. No matter what you hate, you are sure to find at least a couple that you will love. And there are a million really easy ways to cook and season them to bring out all of their flavor. You can find lots of different kinds of vegetables in your supermarket, fresh, frozen, and even organic. If your house is like ours, where we have a tendency to eat the same things over and over, becoming a vegetarian is a good impetus to try something new.

And there's a lot out there. Once yuppies discovered gardening and how to impress their friends with food ("Yes, it's an heirloom yellow tomato that I just discovered. Have you ever tasted anything quite so sweet and juicy?"), farm stands and farmers' markets and local produce stands seemed to take off everywhere. Supermarkets today sell fifteen kinds of lettuce, tropical fruits, celery and celery root, broccoli and broccoli rabe, the most exotic mushrooms, oranges from Spain, and purple potatoes.

> *"If you know the guy who grew it, it's going to taste better."*
>
> —David Page, owner of New York's Home and Drovers Tap Room Restaurants

We know how to cook them, we know how to grow them so they're full of flavor, we know how to get them to the store while they're still fresh and crisp. Let's put it this way: there's never been a better time to be a zucchini.

My advice to you: Dig them. Cultivate them. Get to know them. Vegetables will be your friends. Before we get to what's the difference between a green pepper and a red pepper (a red pepper is just a more mature green pepper that costs more) and how young you have to be to be a new potato (all potatoes are new potatoes when they're dug), here's a few tips that chefs, cooks, and produce people told me over and over. *Buy it fresh. Keep it simple. Don't be intimidated. Fancier doesn't make it better.*

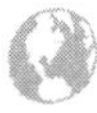

> *"Don't eat anything your ancestors wouldn't have recognized . . . the art of eating has become far too complicated. You can eat 'healthy' foods from the grocery store—like a fat-free, fudge-rolled granola bar that has all the appropriate amounts of protein, vitamins, and minerals—and have a horrible diet. We still don't know all the substances in foods that keep us healthy, but we do know that by simply eating whole foods, with lots of fresh fruits and vegetables, you're covered."*
>
> —Joan Gussow, professor of nutrition at Columbia University Teachers College, quoted by *Health* magazine, May–June 1997

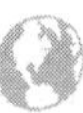

Now my advice on their advice.

Fresh

You can't always buy it fresh; in the middle of February it's awfully hard to find any vegetable, even in the fanciest store, that doesn't look kind of exhausted and saggy. When you can't get it fresh, get something that's a good substitute or don't get it at all. For example, in the winter, to make a terrific tomato sauce buy either plum tomatoes or the Italian canned tomatoes.

And there are times when you just don't want to get fresh—if you don't have the time or patience to clean fresh spinach (true grit and zillions of washings), it's nice to know that plain frozen spinach is quick and tasty.

Aside from buying it fresh, try to buy it organic if you can. Organic foods are less likely to contain pesticide residues and organic farming is less destructive to the environment. Just about everyone I interviewed who cares about food/nutrition/health is a passionate advocate of organic foods. John Gottfried, owner of New York's Gourmet Garage and one of the largest buyers of fine specialty produce in the country, knows the best, cares about quality, and takes a slightly contrary point of view. "By all means, go ahead and buy organic," he advises, "if the quality is the same. But don't think that organic means that some magic wand was waved over it. If you buy any fruit and just wash it really well, you'll be fine."

Keep It Simple

Simple can mean boiled to death in gallons of water (cafeteria food, diners, the army, my mother) or it can mean lightly steamed, then sautéed briefly with a little olive oil and garlic, and sprinkled with a little lemon juice and sea salt. It's the difference between simply awful and simply sensational.

Don't Be Intimidated

The first time I ever cooked (let alone ate) artichokes was in Marcella Hazan's Italian cooking class. If it weren't for that class, I don't think I would ever have known how delicious and easy to cook this vegetable could be. Up until then, I couldn't figure out those step-by-step diagrams of how to chop the leaves and get rid of the choke. It was like trying to figure out how to do brain surgery from pictures. I finally figured it out by watching my friend Donna prepare one. And I saw how straightforward it was. *Don't be intimidated* means "if you don't know what it is, ask." Or just give it a shot—what's the worst that could happen? (Really what's the downside to a slightly undercooked or slightly overcooked artichoke, as long as you get to dip the leaves in a garlic-butter sauce?) If you're not sure how to cook it (or even pronounce it!), see if someone will tell you or show you. If you're curious about how unfamiliar dishes taste, try new stuff in restaurants before you try them at home.

Fancier Doesn't Make It Better

Somewhere along the line we figured out that three vegetables in a rich cream sauce, topped with slivered almonds and melted cheese wasn't superior to one perfectly nice vegetable, like a bunch of matchstick carrots roasted with a little vegetable broth and lemon juice, then miraculously transformed into a glistening and sweetly caramelized dish. Don't disguise flavors—figure out how to bring them out and make them sparkle. And don't think that people will think you didn't try if you don't serve fancy dishes. They'll be more impressed with the perfect simplicity of a dish.

Vegetables

They're incredibly healthy and totally good for you and make your parents deliriously happy when you eat them. Try to overlook all that and like them anyway.

Here's some of my favorites, along with some suggestions for how to cook them. If you are helping make dinner, try a new vegetable or a new technique or a new recipe. Or ask your parents if they will rethink the usual menu and try a vegetable none of you is used to having. They might thank you for introducing them to something wonderful.

> *"How do our children actually stay alive and keep growing since they refuse to eat almost everything? . . . My basic approach is to offer them a variety of healthy and tasty things, then let them do pretty much what they want. (If after three years they have not touched a vegetable, I will go ahead and force them to eat one.)"*
>
> —Anna Thomas, *The New Vegetarian Epicure*

asparagus

Although available throughout the year, asparagus is truly a spring phenomenon. The tips of these green spears should be tight and purplish, the stems fading from green to white and not dried out or fibrous. When you cook them, break off the end of the stem where it naturally snaps in half. You can blanch them, steam them, grill them, roast them, or sauté them. Just don't overcook them. Asparagus loves lemon juice or vinegar and olive oil. (At the risk of seeming indelicate, after you eat asparagus, you'll notice that your urine takes on a vivid green color and smells funny. Vegetable chemistry in action.)

artichokes

You've got to hand it to the Native Americans—they watched lobsters crawling on the beach and figured out that you could actually eat one. Then they figured out how to eat an artichoke. All I can say is, take a look at the pictures in a cookbook or ask someone to show you how to do it. Rub artichokes with lemon juice to keep them from turning brown. Hands down, the easiest way to cook an artichoke is to stand it upright in a saucepan filled with about an inch and a half of boiling water; then cook it for about forty-five minutes, or until the leaves pull out easily. Just be sure to keep an eye on the level of the water. Artichokes can also be deep-fried, braised, and roasted.

To eat an artichoke, scrape your teeth across the base of each leaf, leaf by leaf, until you reach the leaves with the thorny tips that are too tiny and fragile to eat. Now, take a spoon and scrape out those leaves and all the fuzzy interior, called the "choke." You've reached the best part of the artichoke, the heart. Artichokes are great hot or cold, dipped in a vinaigrette, butter and lemon, or a creamy hollandaise sauce.

avocados

Let's put it in perspective: without avocados there would be no guacamole. Without guacamole, there would be no Mexican restaurants or blue corn chips or cobb salad or . . . It's the kind of thing that's so scary you don't want to *think* about it. Avocados are so good you just have to get over the fact that they have tons of calories and are really fattening.

You can get avocados fresh all year. The best kind is the small, dark green-black, pebbly skinned Hass variety. Buy them when they're hard and just let them ripen on the kitchen counter. (If you want to speed up the ripening, put them in a paper bag and close it tight.) Test for ripeness by squeezing—if the flesh gives a little, the fruit is probably ripe. Withered and squishy ones are overripe and shouldn't be eaten. Avocados quickly turn brown when they're cut, so sprinkle lemon juice on them to prevent this.

The other thing that's special about avocados is that each one comes with a free plant. Just put the pit in water, secure it with toothpicks, and wait for it to grow roots. In a couple of weeks you can put it in a pot of soil and watch it grow.

beans

Fresh Beans Fresh summer beans are wonderful (the more snap a bean has, the fresher it is). Just snap off their tips and blanch them (throw them in a big pot with lots and lots of boiling water for just a few minutes) until they are a balance of tender and crisp; then drain and rinse them under really cold water (this keeps them green). Either eat them right away or shorten their cooking time by a few minutes so they remain crisp, and you can finish cooking them later. (They're perfect sautéed in a little olive oil and then spritzed with fresh lemon.)

Wax beans are just yellow string beans. Purple string beans are magic: they turn green when you cook them. Haricots verts are those super-thin French beans you sometimes see in the store. Canned green beans are good if you're eating dinner someplace like the NASA Space Shuttle and you can't stop at the farmers' market. Frozen string beans aren't much better.

Dried Beans Reconstituted dried beans are basic to a good vegetarian diet, but what you can make with them is anything but basic. Hummus, black beans and rice, bean and roasted vegetable burritos, summer bean stew, Tuscan white bean and rosemary puree on pita wedges, black bean chili. On their own, beans can be bland, but it's easy to bring their subtle flavor out. Vegetables add sweetness, garlic and spices add depth, fresh herbs add sparkle, ethnic seasonings add complexity.

There are two kinds of beans you'll be using: the uncooked dried ones and the canned ones. Each has pros and cons. Dried beans are fresher and better textured. The fresher you can get them, the better, so buy them, if you can, at a store that sells lots of beans and has a big turnover. Try health food stores or specialty food stores as opposed to grocery stores. The down side of uncooked dried beans is that, except for split peas and lentils, it's generally recommended that you soak dried beans in water overnight before you cook with them. Soaking helps them cook faster, puts moisture back in, and takes away some of the sugar that causes indigestion. After you soak them, throw out the soaking water, add fresh water, and then boil for about five minutes. Then, finally, you're ready to cook with them. Any vegetarian cookbook will tell you how to prepare each type of bean.

Canned beans are a great time saver (because they're already cooked) but can be kind of mushy and fall apart when you put them into a soup or a stew. The trick to using them is to empty the can into a colander; drain the beans; and then gently rinse off the thick, pasty liquid they come in. Canned chickpeas consistently hold their shape, whereas red kidney beans are notoriously broken and mushy. Frankly, I think if you just want to make a quick dip or burrito filling, go with the canned and you'll be perfectly happy.

Here are some common beans you will probably establish a meaningful relationship with.

Black Beans: Good for soups, stews, and chilis; they love onions, garlic, and tropical fruits.

Cannellini (white kidney-shaped beans): Sublime with olive oil and garlic, good for soups and pasta dishes, can be mashed as dip or spread.

Chickpeas (aka garbanzo beans): Love to be put in the food processor with tahini, garlic, and olive oil; the basis for hummus.

Great Northern Beans (off-white kidney-shaped beans): Good baked, mashed, and pureed; they have an affection for garlic and olive oil.

Kidney Beans (red, white, or pink): Large, sturdy, and filling; good for stews and chili.

Lentils (lots of different colors; split or whole): Cook very quickly, great for soups and stews.

Navy Beans: Smaller version of Great Northerns.

Pinto Beans: Good for mashing; great as refried beans.

Split Peas (green or yellow): Good for soups and sauces.

broccoli

You know how every family has someone in it who's pretty much perfect? Well, that's broccoli, the vegetable most likely to succeed. It's sturdy, reliable, and not the least bit temperamental. It's high in all sorts of nutrients—calcium, vitamin C, and iron—plus it's got cancer-fighting properties. At its best it's lightly steamed; then sautéed with a little garlic or stir-fried with soy sauce and ginger. It's at its worst in salad bars, all those wilted raw florets next to the gloppy dips.

cabbage

Speaking of families, did you know that broccoli is the first cousin of cabbage? (So are Brussels sprouts and cauliflower.) Cabbage is good for making cole slaw and sauerkraut. It's a solid, peasant vegetable, good in soups and stews. If you steam it, you can peel off the leaves and fill them with a vegetable-grain stuffing. Tie each bundle up with baker's twine and bake it.

carrots

Carrots taste better raw than when they're steamed or boiled, but they really shine when roasted or pureed. You can do just about anything to carrots, including juicing. Don't buy them canned or frozen, and watch out for the bags in the supermarket that look like they've been sitting there since the Spanish-American War.

cauliflower

With beautiful creamy white, tightly packed florets surrounded by large green husky leaves, cauliflower has a delicate cabbage flavor. When very fresh, it has a faint scent of cabbage, which led Mark Twain to say, "Cauliflower is just a cabbage with a college education!" Good raw or steamed (in soups or salads), deep-fried (in tempura batter), or mashed with potatoes.

corn

On the cob or off, fresh, frozen, even canned, corn is good. In season, local, just-picked corn is one of the reasons God made summer. And all a fresh ear of corn needs is butter and salt. The fresher it is, the less time it takes to cook. Everyone will tell you that he or she knows the best way to cook corn. And, of course, everyone has a different best way. One of the most charming is related by Bert Greene in his book *Greene on Greens*. He tells about the Shakers, who placed the corn in a pot of cold water and waited for it to boil. Then they covered it and said the Lord's Prayer. When the Lord's Prayer was done, so was the corn.

Corn has inspired lots of American expressions: "that's corny," "corn high," "cornball." In the early 1900s, baseball players called an easy fly ball "a can of corn," because, in that era, grocers stored their canned goods on the higher shelves. To get a can down, the grocer tipped the can forward with a broom handle and caught it.

cucumbers

Regular cucumbers have a thick skin and are waxed (to extend their shelf life), so make sure you peel them with a vegetable peeler. The long cukes you see wrapped in plastic at the store are seedless. The average cucumber has only about ten calories and is mostly water. Cucumbers are great diced up with tomatoes for a refreshing salad in the summer.

eggplant

Eggplant can be a wonderful marriage partner for garlic, onion, cheese, tomatoes, pasta, and herbs. Eggplant Parmigiana anyone? However, on its own, it's kind of bland. Salting and leaving it to drain in a colander removes its bitterness. Beware, it is also like a sponge—eggplant soaks up oil when you're frying it. The trick is to make sure you take all the moisture away before you fry and to get your oil really hot.

garlic

When you're not using it to ward off vampires, you can use garlic to enhance other flavors and to add incredible punch to everything from bread to broccoli. Slice it, mince it, crush it, press it, but don't use too much of it. The whole garlic bulb is called a head, which is separated into cloves. Just the smell of a few cloves of garlic sautéing in a golden olive oil is irresistible. Fresh garlic is so easy to buy and store that there's almost no reason to ever substitute garlic powder, which tastes nothing like fresh. To peel garlic, press the broad side of a knife down firmly on each clove until the paper shell cracks.

greens, sturdy

Just because they sound like they graduated from some vegetable military academy, don't let the name *sturdy* greens scare you. These are all the leafy greens that when young are tender enough to be eaten raw in salads or quickly sautéed with a little oil, but when mature tend to be husky and somewhat tough. These include spinach, chard, beet greens, kale, collard greens, mustard greens, and turnip greens. They are nice in soups; they perk up with a little jolt of garlic and hot red pepper flakes; and most are incredibly high in calcium, potassium, iron, and vitamins.

Eating dark green and yellow orange vegetables may help keep colds and flus at bay. In a recent U.S. Department of Agriculture study, subjects consumed lunches that included five servings of kale and sweet potatoes for three weeks. By one measure, the strength of the participants' immune systems rose 33 percent.

—*Glamour,* June 1997

lettuce

Thanks to yuppies and small farmers and green markets and technology, there is an abundance of choices for making a green salad. Bags of prewashed romaine, Bibb, and mesclun are now in supermarkets year-round. Again, always wash the lettuce—even if the package says the greens are already washed—to remove bacteria. Try something you've never tried before: radicchio, mizuma, or tatsoi. Top with sprouts or roasted nuts or sprinkle with blue cheese. And while supermarket lettuce is never described as tender or innocent or translucent or pure, grow your own and you will find yourself using a whole new vocabulary.

mushrooms

There are dozens of different kinds of mushrooms in America. The only kind you don't want to use are the poisonous ones. (Just a joke.) The most ubiquitous and most popular mushrooms are the small white button variety. They are also the most boring. Mushrooms have a smoky, woodsy flavor; and they're easy to cook and incredibly versatile. One of the best mushrooms for a vegetarian is the meaty (sorry) portobello—it's large enough to stuff or to grill (brushed with olive oil) and makes a great veggie burger (there's a recipe for one in the next chapter). Some mushrooms are sold dried. Their flavor, when reconstituted in water, is deeper and earthier than when fresh. Some great fresh mushrooms to try are chanterelles, cremini, morels, porcini, and shiitakes.

onions

Like garlic, onions are a kitchen essential. Onions make meaningful contributions to soups, salads, pilafs, stews, dips, sauces, sandwiches, pizzas, focaccias, stuffings, stocks, burritos, wraps, and vinaigrettes. And could you imagine a life without onion rings? Definitely not worth living. There are sweet onions, sharp onions, cooking onions, red onions, pearl onions, and even onions that don't seem like onions—shallots and scallions, for instance. The sweetest are Vidalia onions, which are grown in Vidalia, Georgia. How do you know that's where they're from? Well, when a number of Georgia farmers claimed that their fields were the true home of Vidalia onions, a judge had to be called in to settle the dispute. He ruled that only an onion grown within thirty miles of Vidalia could be called a Vidalia.

How to keep from crying when you're cutting onions? Try cutting them under water or chilling them before you cut them. Or you could wear a snorkel mask or ski goggles and completely humiliate yourself.

peas

Like asparagus, peas announce the arrival of spring. Tender, tiny, green, crisp, and unbearably sweet when they are just picked, fresh peas are delicious eaten raw. (Never buy peas that are already shelled.) You can steam, blanch, or sauté fresh peas. You can add them to a pasta primavera. You can make a fresh cream of pea soup. You can add some butter and fresh mint and be happy. If it isn't spring, you can buy frozen peas and pretend.

peppers

There are two kinds of peppers: sweet and chile. The most common sweet pepper is the green pepper, also called the bell pepper. Those red, yellow, and orange peppers you see in the produce section are just fully ripened green peppers—slightly sweeter, slightly more flavorful, and usually more expensive. Chile peppers come in a variety of shapes, colors, sizes, and degrees of heat (one-alarm, two-alarm, three-alarm). Out of two-hundred-odd varieties, a few of the most popular are jalapeños, poblanos, and serranos. A FEW WORDS OF CAUTION: Some chiles are extremely hot. They can burn your fingers, and then anything your fingers subsequently touch, like (ouch!) your eyes. So wear rubber gloves when handling chiles.

potatoes

Potatoes are known by their color: white, purple, red. They're known by their geography: Idaho, Maine, California. They're known by their starch content: new potatoes have low starch, a firm texture, and won't fall apart when you put them in soups and salads; older potatoes are high in starch and are suitable for baking and mashing. They're known by their physical characteristics: round whites, russets, fingerlings, round reds. They're known by what they do: boilers, bakers, all-purpose. They used to be brown and tan, but now that vegetables are chic, they can be as zippy as purple Peruvian or as pretty as buttery yellow Finns. So, even though you can do what you always did with potatoes—mash them, roast them, stuff them with steamed vegetables and top with cheese, make a nice soup, or turn them into a warm potato salad—there is so much more variety, so many more possibilities.

And potatoes are the perfect vegetarian/vegan food. Nice and filling. A great comfort food. Inexpensive. Untemperamental. Easy to cook.

Well, maybe not *that* easy. A recent national telephone survey sponsored by the Idaho Potato Commission found that 46 percent of the one thousand adults polled thought that the best way to bake a potato was to wrap it in foil, like all those steak house–type places do. NO, NO, NO! Putting foil on the potato steams it, makes it moist, and doesn't crisp the skin. The commission recommends baking potatoes at 500°F for forty-five to sixty minutes (depending on size), unwrapped. Prick them a few times with a fork to keep them from exploding while they're baking.

(From Health *magazine, April 1998) On potatoes: "Most of the vitamin C in a potato is in its starchy flesh. But the skin holds 100% of its fiber, potassium, and B vitamins." So eat the skin!*

If you are really crazy about potatoes, you'll be happy to know that Potato Museum, a division of the Food Museum, is online. It features a potato newsletter, potato lore, and even a potato joke of the month. (Why didn't the mother potato want her daughter to marry the famous newscaster? *Are you sitting down?* Because he was a commontater.) *All this and more at www.foodmuseum.com/~hughes/first.htm.*

sea vegetables

Sea vegetables are an excellent source of protein, vitamins, and minerals. Asian cultures traditionally use sea vegetables in their cuisine. Probably the most familiar to us is nori, paper-thin sheets of seaweed traditionally used to wrap the sticky rice in sushi rolls. Some other sea vegetables you might encounter are dulse, a deep-red leafy vegetable that's good in soups and stews; kombu, which is dehydrated kelp; and wakame, dehydrated kelp that's more delicate and milder tasting than kombu. Both kombu and wakame are traditionally used in miso soup.

As a bizarre aside, I once had a rental car for three days whose interior smelled mysteriously like nori (kind of sweet and salty). The smell was so alluring that for three nights in a row, on my way home from work, I stopped in at my favorite Japanese restaurant and stuffed myself on big platters of sushi. (No, it wasn't a Japanese car.)

squash

There are two kinds of squash: thick-skinned winter squash (like acorn, butternut, and turban) and thin-skinned summer squash (like zucchini, yellow squash, and pattypan). When you're buying summer squash, the smaller the better—fewer seeds, less water, more flavor. Cook these delicate vegetables with fresh herbs, olive oil, tomatoes, cheese, onions, or pasta. They're nice braised or sautéed. Try not to soak or boil summer squash, because they're watery to begin with and they'll get kind of soggy. Winter squash have a richer, sweeter flavor than summer squash and the word *delicate* doesn't begin to apply to these magnificent hulks. With winter squash, the bigger the better. And you can keep them in a cool place for months and months without them suffering any adverse effects. You can boil or braise or simply bake them, kind of like potatoes. After they're cooked, you can squash them and mix them with a little salt, butter, and cream (or brown sugar, my favorite). How can you not like a vegetable that's both a noun and a verb?

tomatoes

Generally speaking, there are only two kinds of tomatoes worth eating. The first kind is any summer tomato that's garden grown, just picked, sweet, sun ripened, juicy, and aromatic. These can be big red beefsteak tomatoes, classic slicing tomatoes, thicker-skinned plum tomatoes, or tiny yellow or crimson cherry tomatoes. No matter what the size is, they're all bursting with flavor. And you can do anything to them (including nothing except slice and sprinkle them with some sea salt), and they will go from superb to sublime. The only thing you shouldn't do to them is to refrigerate them—just store them at room temperature or keep them in a cool place.

In the winter, pretty much abandon all hope. Your choices tend to be those rocklike, juiceless, pale red tomatoes that are in a perpetual state of chemical unripeness; wildly expensive hydroponic tomatoes; okay-tasting and pricey imported tomatoes; and occasionally passable plum tomatoes.

Which brings us to the second kind of really good tomatoes: canned tomatoes. It sounds unlikely, but this is one canned product that's really excellent. Whole peeled plum tomatoes are the most versatile kind; serve them stewed (dump the contents of the can in a saucepan, bring to a simmer with a little butter and/or olive oil, season with salt and pepper) or slice, crush, dice, or puree as needed. The simplest tomato sauce in the world uses a can of tomatoes, a little garlic, a little extra-virgin olive oil, and some salt and pepper.

It's fun to grow your own tomatoes and you've got some great varieties to pick from. I love names like Ponderosa Red, Pink Odoriko (yes, it's Japanese), Mr. Stripey, Subarctic Plenty, Hybrid Celebrity, Hybrid Miracle Sweet. My new favorite is a huge four-pounder the seed company calls Mortgage Lifter. But take it from me, there's a reason God made farm stands and green markets. Two summers ago, I asked my green-thumbed husband if he would grow tomatoes. He put in about ten plants and took great care of them. But between the deer, the heat, the rain, the mildew, the moles, and the slugs, all we wound up with in mid-August was one edible tomato. Which, I figured, totaling all the expenses involved, probably cost us about $75.00.

Fruit

To every fruit (turn, turn, turn) there is a season (turn, turn, turn). Although lots of fruits are available year-round (bananas, grapes, oranges, lemons), most have seasons during which they really shine. The difference between a summer strawberry and a winter strawberry is astounding. So, like vegetables, when you can buy local and seasonal and organic fruit, do so. And although a plate of fresh fruit might not seem like a big treat, there are nice, simple things you can do to make fruit more appealing (fruit compotes, applesauce, fruit cobblers, poached fruits).

> *A British long-term study of the relationship of diet to health in eleven thousand vegetarians and other health-conscious people found that participants lived longer than the general population. In the study, one factor stood out: Those who ate fresh fruit every day lived longer and were less likely to die from a heart attack or stroke.*
>
> —*Glamour,* June 1997

Herbs

Dried herbs are fine in a pinch (no pun intended), but like everything else in the vegetable world, if they're fresh, they're better. And it's easier than ever now to get fresh herbs year-round, prepackaged in local supermarkets. However, if dry is all that is available, keep in mind that dried herbs are more pungent than fresh, so you need to use only one teaspoon of the dried herb as opposed to two or three teaspoons of the fresh herb.

Grains

Grains are everything from couscous to barley to rice to kamut to corn. The form grains take range from whole grains (like oats and barley) to milled grains (like flour). And grain is *everything* to many people and many cultures. Half of the world population's main sustenance, for example, is rice. The rule of thumb is, the more refined and processed the grain, the less taste, texture, and nutritional value. Thus whole wheat flour, for example, is better for you than processed white flour.

Although supermarkets carry a large variety of grains, you'll probably find a better selection at health food or whole food stores, which sell in bulk and sell a lot. Store grains in tightly covered glass jars in a cool place. Some grains are more perishable than others; and generally, the more refined the grain, the longer the shelf life. If you're not sure, ask.

Let's put the cards on the table. Most grains do not have a lot of appeal. Really, how appealing could a grain like millet be, when most of us know it as birdseed? And does "cornmeal mush" sound like something you can't wait to come home to? Plain brown rice, all by itself, is about as dreary as food can get outside of prison. So the goal is to jazz it up, give it a little color and contrast and zip. Seasoning the cooking liquid with spices and adding chopped vegetables and herbs, dried fruit, or even canned tomatoes with lots of juice are some easy ways to add interest. Here are some grains worth knowing.

barley

Barley comes in a variety of forms, but pearl barley is the most common and easy to prepare. It requires no soaking and cooks in about thirty minutes. It's good in soups like mushroom barley, but you can also serve it as a substitute for rice.

buckwheat

Buckwheat, in spite of its name, is actually a fruit. But because it doesn't act like a fruit, we treat it like a grain. Go figure. Whole, untoasted buckwheat groats are known as kasha. Traditionally used with egg noodles in the Jewish dish kasha varnishkes, buckwheat has a strong, deep, nutty flavor that's good for soups and stews.

bulgur

Wheat berries that have been hulled, steamed, roasted, and cracked are known as bulgur. Milled into three different textures, bulgur cooks up very quickly. The most common bulgur is the tiny grain you see flecked throughout the Middle Eastern parsley-tomato salad called tabbouleh.

corn

Corn is the only grain we eat as a fresh vegetable. But we also eat it dried and ground in dishes like cornbread; muffins; corn tortillas; and cornmeal mush, which the Italians are smart enough to call "polenta." Traditional polenta takes about forty-five minutes to cook; but you can buy instant polenta, which is a good substitute, that takes only about ten minutes.

couscous

Couscous is to North Africa what rice is to the Far East. The mild flavor of this delicate grain absorbs the flavors it's cooked with. Traditionally, it's steamed and served with stewed meats or vegetables. Couscous is available in a quick-cooking form that just needs to be soaked in hot liquid and fluffed with a fork. Beware the boxed quick-cooking flavored couscous—the flavors tend to taste stale and artificial. It's easy enough to add your own flavorings.

oats

Whole-grain oats are great for adding to muffins and bread, but oats are truly terrific in the guise of that old favorite oatmeal. There's lots of different kinds of oatmeal, but even the instant packages make a great, quick hot breakfast. Try using apple juice in place of water when you cook it—it makes the oatmeal a little sweeter so you'll use less sugar as a topping.

up-and-coming grains

Quinoa: Good luck trying to figure out from looking at it how to pronounce it (it's *keen'wah*). First cultivated by the ancient Incas in the South American Andes, this tiny grain is light, tasty, easy to cook, and incredibly nutritious.

Amaranth: Also a nutrition powerhouse, amaranth is crunchy, sweet, and tasty. It's great as a breakfast cereal, a pudding, or as a thickener for soups and stews. Amaranth, too, was a staple for the Inca Indians.

Teff: A tiny grain that dates back to the ancient Egyptians. It's good as a breakfast cereal or mixed with other grains.

Rice

In many cultures, rice is a mainstay. People who live in China and Japan consume, on average, 330 pounds of rice a year. Incredibly, there are over seven thousand varieties grown around the world. White rice is the most popular grain in the United States, but no matter what the variety, in this country we eat only about 11 pounds per person. There are so many different types of rice worth trying. Following are some of the rices commonly available in your supermarket. For a larger selection, check out health food stores or East Indian and Asian grocery stores. Go to ethnic restaurants and see what's indigenous to different cultures.

brown rice

There are three types of brown rice: short, medium, and long grain. Brown rice is rich in fiber, is nutty in flavor, and has a chewy texture. It takes a lot longer to cook than white rice. It has a short shelf life, though—only about a month—and should be stored in the refrigerator.

white rice

There are three types of white rice: short, medium, and long grain. Medium- and, particularly, short-grain rices are very glutinous, so they're perfect for making Japanese "sticky rice." Cooked long-grain rice is fluffy and separates easily. White rice cooks in about half the time of brown rice—about twenty minutes; and if that's too long, there's even instant rice, which takes only five minutes. Unfortunately, what it adds in convenience it loses in taste: instant rice tends to have mushier, less flavorful kernels. (Instant rice has the dubious distinction of being the least nourishing, least flavorful, and most expensive form of rice.)

One very popular white rice is converted (which sounds like it used to be Jewish but decided to become Catholic). Converted rice is steamed and pressure-cooked before it's milled, which results in a higher vitamin content than regular milled rice. It's also enriched.

wild rice

In spite of its name, it isn't wild (it used to be) and it isn't rice (it's the seed of a water grass). (Wild rice really should be introduced to buckwheat, the fruit that thinks it's a grain.) Wild rice is native to the Great Lakes region of North America. Its long, slender, burnished black-brown kernels produce a rice with a really distinctive flavor—intensely nutty and chewy. Because it's traditionally harvested by hand, it's usually much more expensive than other varieties of rice.

other rices to try

Arborio: An Italian medium-grain rice, pearly white and nearly round, arborio has an enormous capacity to absorb liquid—nearly three times that of regular white rice. This is the rice most often used to make the creamy Italian rice dish risotto. It works well for rice puddings, too.

Basmati: A long-grain white or brown rice from India, known for its fluffy texture and distinctive floral aroma. The grain actually lengthens when cooked. Although brown basmati is more nutritious, it hasn't nearly the flavor or aroma of the white basmati.

Jasmine: Another subtly fragrant long-grain white rice, Jasmine rice was originally from Thailand. It remains moist and tender, but not fluffy, when cooked properly.

Pasta

The miracle of pasta is that from essentially three humble ingredients (flour, water, egg—and you don't even have to use all three) practically a whole new food group is created. Only two ingredients, flour and water, are used to make all the dry varieties you get in the grocery store, like spaghetti, linguine, macaroni, and penne. Homemade pasta, or fresh pasta—like ravioli and tortellini—is made with eggs and flour. Which is better? Dry pasta is terrific once you find a good brand (Ronzoni and DeCecco are excellent). And fresh egg pasta is great when it's really fresh and homemade but truly terrible when it's not.

What's so good about pasta? You mean beside the fact that you can cook it in no time, without lifting a finger? Or that it's so incredibly adaptive and versatile? Or that by adding different kinds of vegetables and herbs, and sauces and broths, you can create enormous numbers of sensational dishes? Oh nothing really, I suppose. You can sauce it, stuff it, bake it, eat it hot or cold, enjoy it winter or summer. It's inexpensive, accessible, universally liked, and deeply satisfying. Put it this way: if pasta were a person, you would marry it.

Some tips. Don't ever rinse cooked pasta in cold water after you drain it—the sauce won't stick if the pasta is cool. Use lots and lots of water when you cook it so the pasta has room to move around. Homemade pasta, by the way, cooks in a minute or two, tops. Dried pastas take ten to twelve minutes—taste to see if it's *al dente,* which means "firm to the bite." Most colored pastas look pretty but taste a little weird; the color is more of a gimmick than a flavor. Speaking of flavor, don't ever use the Parmigiano-Reggiano cheese you can buy in a jar, unless you like the taste of sawdust.

A General Guide to Pasta and Noodle Shapes, Sizes, and Uses

Small Shapes

cavatelli: Shaped like cloud shells; good for chunky sauces.
conchiglie or shells: Shaped like seashells; good for sauces with small chunks; small seashells are good in soups.

farfalle (or bow ties): Shaped like bow ties or butterflies; good for chunky sauces.
fusilli: Shaped like a corkscrew; good for sauces with a big flavor and small chunks.
orecchiette: Shaped like little caps or ears; good for chunky sauces.
ravioli: Shaped into small squares; stuffed with any number of fillings, most commonly cheese; homemade or specialty-store ravioli are best; good with delicate sauces, tomato sauces, or chunky sauces.

Tubes

penne: Shaped like small quills or pencil points; good hot or cold or baked with chunky or smooth sauce.
rigatoni: Shaped like short grooved tubes; good for really bold-flavored sauces.
ziti: Shaped like long thin tubes; good for bold sauces and baked.

Long and Flat Shapes

capelli d'angelo (or angel hair): Shaped into very fine, thin strands; delicate; cooks very quickly; soaks up a ton of sauce; good for light sauces only.
fettuccine: Shaped into long, flat wide strands; particularly good with cream sauces and thick sauces.
lasagne: Shaped into very wide, flat strands; has smooth or ruffled edges; good baked with sauce (in your favorite lasagna).
linguine: Shaped into thin, flat strands; good with medium-thick sauces.
spaghetti: Shaped into thin, round strands; the numbers indicate the thickness of the noodle; good for light to medium-thick sauces.
vermicelli: Shaped into thin, round strands; good with smooth to medium chunky sauces.

Of course, Italians aren't the only noodle aficionados. Asians have been eating noodles for centuries and are something of experts on the subject.

Asian Noodles

bean thread noodles or cellophane noodles: Very thin, long, slippery, translucent noodles typically used in Thai cooking. *Super* easy to prepare; just soak in hot water to soften, drain, and add to soup or use in place of rice with stir-fry.
ramen: Japan's version of Italy's spaghetti and China's mein (as in lo mein). As good as the quick-cooking packages of ramen noodles taste, you should know that they're loaded with fat and sodium. You can now find baked ramen in the supermarket, which still has quite a bit of sodium but much less fat.
rice noodles or rice stick noodles or rice vermicelli: All made from rice flour and water. These noodles are thin; flat; translucent; and good for stir-fries, soups, and salads. Rice noodles do need to soak in cold water before they're cooked briefly in boiling water.
soba: Japanese buckwheat noodles, which are traditionally served cold. They have a very earthy flavor that takes a little getting used to.
somen: Japan's version of Italy's angel hair pasta. Very thin and delicate; good in broth with steamed vegetables or cold with a dipping sauce.
udon: Thick white or whole wheat noodles. Udon noodles are most often available flat, like fettuccine, but also come round. Good in soups, stews, and casseroles.

Oils

All vegetable oils contain the same number of calories (120 calories per tablespoon) and the same amount of fat (fourteen grams per tablespoon). One difference is how they're made. (Is the oil polyunsaturated, monounsaturated, or saturated? Is it very bad for you, not too bad, or actually okay in moderation?) And, of course, a big difference is how they all taste. Somehow, if you balance something you like the taste of with something that won't give you a heart attack, you will find an oil you can cook with and an oil you can use for salad dressing.

Butter and the so-called *tropical oils*—coconut, palm, and palm kernel—are all saturated fats. Generally, saturated fats (the academic nutrition journals I read refer to them as "sat fats") are the ones to steer clear of. They clog your arteries, give you heart attacks, and make you jiggle. The best use of butter is to use in small amounts with olive oil when you are sautéing. The butter gives your food a nice, creamy flavor and the oil keeps the butter from burning.

Corn, safflower, and *sunflower oils* are polyunsaturated fats. They are mild enough to be good all-purpose cooking oils.

Olive, canola, and *peanut oils* are monounsaturated fats. Canola is low in saturated fat, is mild, and has just enough flavor to enhance the foods cooked with it—all of which has made it a popular oil with people concerned about health and taste. Olive oil, whether a rich, fruity green or a lush gold is a delicious, full-bodied choice, regardless if you're sautéing or making a salad dressing. Olive oils are touted as far better for you than other oils, the proof being that they are the main oil in the Mediterranean diet, which is exceptionally healthy. There are great olive oils imported from Spain and Italy and some wonderful California olive oils. Try lots of different kinds and see what you like best.

One of the best innovations (all the chefs I interviewed love them) are the spray cooking oils. Coat the pan you'll be cooking in and use only the smallest amount of oil. That way you get all the flavor with very few calories.

Oil Trivia

Canola oil sounds like it might come from a nut or berry or field in Iowa, right? A natural kind of oil with a natural name? Think again. The name *canola* was made up by the Canadian company that developed the oil. The *Can* in the name is for "Canada." The *ol* is for "oil." The *a* is to give the word a flourish. Canola oil is actually rapeseed oil, fat from the seeds of the mustard plant.

Vinegars

There are a few basic types of vinegars, and then there are all the fancy fruit-flavored ones (like raspberry and blueberry) and the ones in the pretty bottles filled with herbs (that sometimes start to look like weeds in a matter of weeks) that the neighbors give your parents at Christmas. What's what?

Balsamic Vinegar

At first, American cooks liked this dark amber Italian vinegar because it adds so much zing and an almost-sweet splash to grilled vegetables, tofu, and marinades. This vinegar doesn't just dress a salad—it invigorates it. Then balsamic vinegar became trendy, and everyone used it for everything. Then, because it was so trendy, lots of wannabe balsamic vinegars came on the market, which bore almost no resemblance to the real thing. So *do* use balsamic vinegar, *don't* use it on *everything* and make sure it's authentic.

Balsamic Vinegar: The best is rich and almost syrupy; a kind of balance between sweet and tangy; quite expensive because it's been aged and mellowed.

Cider Vinegar: The color of apple juice with a slight apple or fruit taste; particularly good in cole slaw.

Fruit-flavored Vinegar: Light and lovely; nice mixed with olive oil on a field salad or splashed alone on a fruit salad.

Herb Vinegar: Can perk up an otherwise boring salad. Ditto on cooled vegetables.

Red Wine Vinegar: Rosy and tangy; a good staple; one of the best vinegars for mixing with olive oil (a traditional vinaigrette) for a splendid salad dressing.

Rice Wine Vinegar: An Asian vinegar; light and only mildly acidic; good for light vinaigrettes, dipping sauces, and marinades.

White Vinegar: Clear and colorless; very astringent; good for pickling and dyeing your Easter eggs (it is different from white wine vinegar).

White Wine Vinegar: Pale and nicely tart; a good staple for salad dressings, marinades, and sauces.

Soy Products

Soy products are so good for you (soybeans have more protein and calcium than other legumes), you just have to figure out how to be good to them. "Tofu," says an eighteen-year-old vegetarian I know who likes good food, "always tastes better when I eat out." When I related this mystery to Deborah Madison, the guru of vegetarian cooking, she didn't chuckle like I thought she would. "That's probably because when she eats out, she's eating tofu in Japanese or Chinese restaurants, where it is such an integral part of the cuisine," Ms. Madison says. "It just tastes right as part of certain dishes."

So don't think of soy products (like I tend to) as mysterious ingredients to be wrestled with because they're good for you and don't just throw them into any old dish to add protein. Try to give them time and the benefit of the doubt (Phoebe hated soy milk when she first started drinking it and now loves the taste), and do try soy products in ethnic restaurants or great health food restaurants so you know how good they can taste.

miso

Miso is fermented soybean paste. It is most commonly used to make a traditional Japanese soup.

soy milk

Soy milk is made from cooked, ground soybeans. It's rich in protein; but unless it's fortified, it lacks the calcium of cow's milk. It can be used in all recipes calling for milk.

tempeh

Tempeh is fermented, split, cooked soybeans, which are then pressed into cakes. It is an Indonesian staple and has a tender, chewy taste and a nutty, robust flavor. It's good marinated and grilled, stir-fried, baked, and added to stews and chili as a substitute for meat.

tofu

Tofu has been part of Chinese cooking since 200 B.C. It's a food that's still essential to the Asian diet. Tofu is made from the curds of coagulated soy milk, which are pressed into blocks. These blocks can be very firm or as soft as a full-bodied custard. Tofu is a major source of protein and iron and other vitamins and minerals. By itself, it's kind of bland. But when it absorbs the flavors that it's cooking with (a Thai coconut sauce, a sesame marinade, a curried carrot soup), this plain, nondescript food turns into something amazing. It's kind of the Cinderella of soy foods.

Tofu needs to be refrigerated and used within a week (or less), because it's very perishable. Keep it in water and change the water every day. If it starts to smell funny, throw it out. You can also freeze tofu for up to three months; freezing gives it a chewier texture. Tofu is available in four textures, and recipes will usually tell you which type of tofu to use.

The Aliens

Laura Boggs, a fourteen-year-old vegetarian from Albany, New York, describes her first experience with a tofu pup: "It was hard on the outside, gooey on the inside. You can't kill them. If you put them in the microwave too long they bounce when you take them out. One bite and I was sick."

Extra-Firm and Firm: Particularly good for grilling or cubing and using in stir-fries, soups, and stews. You can also crumble it to make scrambled tofu. This is the best choice of tofu if you are making a dish for which you want the tofu to retain its shape.

Soft: More tender and delicate with a higher water content than firm tofu. Because it can become kind of creamy, it lends itself to salad dressings and sauces, and fruit shakes.

Silken: This variety has the most delicate consistency and works best in blended or pureed recipes, like frostings and puddings.

tvp

Textured vegetable protein is soy flour in the form of granules. TVP is sold in a dehydrated form; after you add boiling water, it takes on a chewy consistency like ground beef. *The Vegetarian Way* calls TVP, "a wonderful food made from soy protein." Deborah Madison in her book *Vegetarian Cooking for Everyone* calls it, "a sawdustlike by-product used to replace meat." You make the call.

Nonsoy Meat Substitute: Seitan

In a category of its own, seitan is for the dedicated vegetarian who misses the texture of meat. Made from high-protein wheat flour, seitan is wheat gluten. Rich in protein, low in fat, with a chewy texture and mild flavor, this gluten can be baked and used as a meat substitute. You can find it dried (it needs to be rehydrated) or already prepared (in the refrigerator section). It's often called "wheat meat."

The Problem With Tofu Is . . .

(An Unenlightened Look at Health Food)

To me, foreign food isn't French or Italian or Japanese. It's sprouts and rice milk and soy flour and dehydrated black bean flakes and things like an eggless mayonnaise sold in health food stores (called Nayonnaise).

I guess it's that kind of skeptical middle-aged attitude that is keeping me from evolving to a higher plane on the vegetarian food chain. That and the fact that I still can't help believing that there is some weird correlation between the fact that the unhealthiest looking people are often the very same ones who wind up working in health food stores. And frankly—I know it's politically incorrect to even bring this up—in our local health food store, these people don't just appear unhealthy, they seem unhappy to boot. Just ask for a bag to put all your stuff in, and they'll roll their eyes like you've just single-handedly destroyed the rain forest.

Maybe it's just that they know I'm not a fellow traveler when they see me in the aisles suspiciously eyeing some wilted organic celery or trying to figure out what you're supposed to do with a pouch of powdered sea kelp. Of course, even the most basic vegetarian ingredients still seem mysterious to me.

I'm not even comfortable with tofu. I know it's Chinese and ancient and one of the most remarkably versatile foods on the planet. But it's white and it jiggles. It doesn't seem like a food. It sounds like it should be a Greek island next to Corfu. It looks weird. It's got a funny name. Except for kung fu and snafu, I can't think of anything, certainly no food, that ends with fu. Anyway, it has more in common with goldfish than with food—you have to change its water every day to keep it fresh. I know it's incredibly adaptable, except I can never figure out what to do with it. For something so completely natural, it doesn't seem natural at all. Jell-O jiggles, and we all love Jell-O; maybe tofu needs a spokesman. Someone jolly like Rosie O'Donnell. Or perky like Cameron Diaz.

And while we're at it, there are other vegetarian foods that could use a little spin control. When I think of wheat germ, I keep getting stuck on the "germ" part of it, and germs make you sick, not healthy. Tempeh, the cultured soybean product, sounds more like a resort in Arizona than a food. And I keep confusing TVP, which stands for textured vegetable protein, with either STP or MVP. Seitan, a natural meat substitute, has the unfortunate coincidence of being pronounced like *Satan*. Spirulina sounds like a lesser-known pasta shape or worse yet, some incurable virus. As in, "She couldn't drink the water in Belize because she was afraid of spirulina."

What else could profit from a more user-friendly name? Well, certainly mung beans, adzuki beans, garbanzo beans, kamut, natto, yuba, spelt, sucanat, triticale. Oh, and wakame, a leafy sea vegetable that sounds like the name of the Girl Scout camp I went to on the eastern shore of Maryland.

Let's face it. At fifty-one, I'm tofu challenged, kelp sensitive, and natto phobic with a slight allergic reaction to health food stores. But I'm more willing than ever to give peas a chance.

P.S.: And one more thing that's confusing. I can't get over the number of vegetarian dishes and recipes that attempt to look just like or taste just like something you don't want to eat in the first place. Like tofu patties, tofu pups, tofu orange "duck," soy "sausage," barbecued gluten "ribs," Breakfast Fakin' Bacon, Foney Baloney, tempeh reubans, unturkey. And the ultimate thrill of the grill, Not Dogs. Which I guess you could top with Nayonnaise.

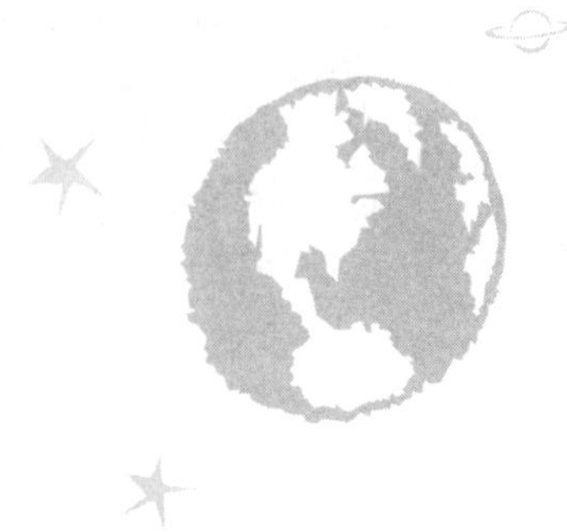

An Enlightened Look at Health Food
by Phoebe

When I started out as a vegetarian, I lived on French fries, pizza, and Sprite. Occasionally, a salad. When I wanted to be healthy I would have some water. I was doing it for all the right reasons (i.e., not because it was trendy); but since then, I've evolved, if you will. I was lacto-ovo for two years, then became vegan. Becoming vegan limited my intake of "normal" foods, cutting out things like pizza and French dressing; so I needed to find more creative ways of eating. Second, I realized that being vegan isn't just a diet . . . it's a way of life. The girl who inspired me to become vegan, Isabel, said that we should be proud of what we put into our bodies, and that really made me think. I went in with an open mind and tried scrambled tofu and tempeh curry and found that I loved it. It gives me the coolest feeling when I'm eating rice in a dark little restaurant with chopsticks or granola and soy milk at a café in SoHo or a wee dragon bowl at Angelica Kitchen in the East Village . . . much more creative than McDonald's, I'd say.

Tofu. My God. (Goddess?) Tofu is amazing. My mother wouldn't say so, though. She's been good, she's tried it; but in that department, I've had to educate my mother more than she's had to educate me.

I could live on tofu. It's so versatile—scrambled tofu for breakfast, baked tofu sandwich for lunch, curried tofu and rice for dinner, and chocolate devastation cake (vegan, of course, made with tofu powder) for dessert. I don't eat it as a substitute for meat or eat it because it's the next best thing to meat. I eat it because I love it!

My mother has been open to tofu, but with a certain amount of skepticism. I understand that it's hard to be introduced to something completely new after fifty-one years of one way of thinking, so maybe she's coming in with as much of an open mind as is possible for her. Figuring out why Phish (the band) spells their name with a *ph* is about as far as she's gotten. It's a start, I guess. Yet her idea of tasting scrambled tofu is taking a fork, sticking it into the bowl, and barely licking the tip of the tines. The way I figure it, we'll start with baby steps and work our way up to whole bites; and before you can say *tofutempehseitan*, she'll be devouring home-style bean curd at the local Chinese restaurant.

chapter 5

★ ★ ★ ★ ★

Recipes

"Keep it simple," says Mollie Katzen, creator of The Moosewood Cookbook. *"When I was a younger cook, I used to think that the more ingredients I could throw in, the more creative the recipe was . . . the best meals are the simplest."*

—*Health* magazine, May–June 1996

When I first started looking for vegetarian recipes and menus and food ideas for our family after Phoebe became a vegetarian (then vegan), I was struck by the fact that some cookbook recipes were really complicated, some were really time-consuming, some called for a whole pantryful of ethnic ingredients that we didn't have access to (even in a suburb of New York City) and weren't sure we really wanted to stock up on. But the recipes that were least appealing were the ones, mostly in vegetarian brochures and newsletters, written specifically for teenagers. No wonder. These recipes weren't written by chefs, restaurant people, cookbook authors, or food people. Almost all of them were written by nutritionists and dieticians.

They were relentlessly earnest and plain. They never seemed like fun. They didn't sound delicious. At the bottom of the recipe (sometimes longer than the recipe itself) were all the nutritional data, calories along with fat and vitamin content. You knew if you made one of these recipes you would be a healthy person. Only I don't think you would be a very happy person.

So all the recipes in this chapter are guaranteed (or your money back) to make you happy and full and satisfied and wish you'd made more. They were all contributed by people who just love food; who love to cook; who love to eat; whose goals in life are to show you all the possibilities of food and to make you practically swoon from a bite, a taste, an aroma. So I guess if it comes down to a choice between nutrition and passion, I'd chose passion every time.

These recipes are an introduction to how good vegetarian food can be, in its infinite variety. They will also introduce you to some of this country's most creative chefs and best-loved restaurants, all of which you can revisit on your own. Eat at Matthew Kenney's Monzu or Angelica Kitchen when you're in New York City, order some incredible raspberry jam from Larry Forgione's American Spoon Foods catalog (the address is in the "Resources" section), watch Chris Schlesinger and John Willougby on the TV Food Network.

When researching this book, I read and studied hundreds and hundreds of cookbooks. There are lots of wonderful books, but there are two I would suggest you buy now. They'll both be dog-eared from use in a matter of months. They're Deborah Madison's *Vegetarian Cooking for Everyone* and the new *Joy of Cooking.* Oddly enough, a recent food article in *The New York Times* referred to *Vegetarian Cooking for Everyone* as the vegetarian *Joy of Cooking.* I agree. Both books are smart and encyclopedic (without being endlessly tedious) and helpful and sensible about food. And the recipes are well written, easy to follow, and delicious.

Enjoy all the recipes that follow. I would love to hear from you if there's something that came out really great or that you had a question or suggestion about. Write me care of Bantam Books, 1540 Broadway, New York, NY 10036. Or send e-mail to Phoebe at xsoygrlx@aol.com. Don't call me collect at 3:00 A.M. with a question about curry powder even if it's a *really* urgent question. My husband needs seven hours of sleep.

> *"The best thing anyone ever said about my cooking is that it's vegetarian but you wouldn't know it."*
>
> —Martha Rose Shulman, *Health* magazine, May–June 1996

Some Tips Before You Start

1. Figure out how to use the food processor and all the different blades. You'll use it a lot.
2. No matter what anyone tells you, there is an enormous amount of prep work in vegetarian cooking—tons of washing and dicing and chopping and soaking and mincing and marinating. Listen to some great music and get into a groove while you do it or do it with a friend to make it feel less daunting.
3. Read a recipe carefully. Do all the chopping, washing, measuring, etc. mentioned in the ingredient list first. That way you won't be surprised in the middle of cooking something when you see you were supposed to chop the peppers or mince the garlic.
4. When you are cutting fresh chiles, remember to wear latex gloves like in *E.R.* so the chiles don't burn your skin.
5. Remember that with baking, you have to be precise or the recipe won't work (the cake won't rise, the dough will be tough) but with cooking, once you master the recipe, you can take liberties. Throw in twice as much basil, use vegetable stock instead of water, add tons more lemon to a hummus or a salad dressing.
6. Make sure your knives are sharp.
7. For things like lentil soup and marinara sauce, as long as you're doing one recipe, you might as well double it and freeze half.

8. Wear short sleeves or roll up your sleeves when you're cooking. Don't cook in bare feet, in case you drop a knife. Long, curly hair is nice on your head, but not in your soup. Pull it back. Don't wear a long flowing scarf around your neck or you might cook yourself.
9. Okay, maybe it's because I'm a middle-aged mother, but you might want to think about wearing an apron.
10. If you follow only one piece of advice, here's the one that separates a happy cook from a miserable, cranky one: Clean as you go.

All recipes for vegans—which have no poultry or dairy at all—are marked with this symbol: (v).

Best Vegetarian Cookbook Title: *The Soy of Cooking*

Most Politically Incorrect Restaurant Name: *Fin & Hoof in Alexandria, Virginia. Their slogan is "Serious Steaks. Serious Seafood. Serious Fun."*

Most Unlikely Cookbook Title: *Betty Crocker's Vegetarian Cookbook*

★ ★ ★ ★ ★

Guacamole (v)

Recipe courtesy Josefina Howard,
Rosa Mexicano, from *Saveur* magazine

makes 1 to 2 cups

Besides using guacamole as a dip, try it in a flour tortilla with some shredded cheese and refried beans. It's incredibly delicious and incredibly versatile.

- 1/4 cup finely chopped white onion
- 1 jalapeño pepper, seeded and minced
- 1 tablespoon finely chopped cilantro
- 1/2 teaspoon salt or more to taste
- 1 medium Hass avocado
- 1 small tomato, coarsely chopped

1. Combine half the onion, half the jalapeño, and half the cilantro in a blender; season with the salt, and blend into a smooth paste. Transfer to a serving bowl.
2. Cut the avocado in half lengthwise; then remove and discard the pit. Make crosshatched incisions in the avocado pulp with a paring knife. Scoop the pulp out with a spoon, and add it to the onion mixture. Mix well with a wooden spoon.
3. Stir in the remaining onion, jalapeño, and cilantro; then gently mix in the tomato. Adjust the seasoning with salt and serve immediately.

Easiest Marinara Sauce
(V, if made without butter)

Melissa Hamilton

Melissa Hamilton is a lifelong foodie with most impressive credentials. Melissa owns a restaurant in Lambertville, New Jersey (Hamilton's Grill Room), had her own catering company, is a frequent contributor to Cooks Illustrated, *does professional food styling, and is currently the head of the test kitchen at* Saveur *magazine. In her spare time, she attempts to convince her two young daughters to eat anything green.*

sauces 1 pound cooked pasta, about 3 cups

This is your basic, year-round, no-fail, always-terrific tomato sauce. It's perfect with any kind of pasta.

- 1/4 cup extra-virgin olive oil
- 1 tablespoon unsalted butter (optional)
- 2 medium garlic cloves, finely minced or pressed through a garlic press
- One 28-ounce can diced tomatoes
- 2 tablespoons chopped fresh basil, parsley, or thyme leaves; or 1 teaspoon dried (optional)
- Salt and freshly milled black pepper

Heat the oil, butter (if using), and garlic together in a medium heavy-bottomed saucepan over medium heat. When the garlic is fragrant, add the tomatoes. Cook, stirring occasionally, until the sauce is the desired thickness, 5 to 10 minutes. Stir in the basil, if desired. Season to taste with salt and pepper.

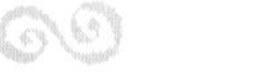  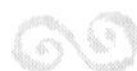

Ultra Tomatoes (v)

Rozanne Gold
Recipes 1–2–3 (Viking, 1996)

Rozanne Gold, a New York chef, figured out that you could make wonderful recipes using just a few ingredients, if you used the right ingredients to maximize flavor. Then she wrote a bunch of very successful "1–2–3" cookbooks, in which all the recipes call for only three ingredients. It sounds kind of gimmicky, but once you cook from her books, you realize that it really works.

Here are two methods for maximizing the flavor of tomatoes. The slow evaporation of the moisture gives even boring tomatoes a sweet, bright, intense taste. The trick is to cook them forever at a very low temperature. Essentially, the oven does all the work. Use these tomatoes to top pizza or pasta, chop them to make salsa, or add them to a bean salad.

I. Slow-Roasted Romas

makes 24 pieces

12 roma (plum) tomatoes, halved lengthwise
3 tablespoons extra-virgin olive oil
3 garlic cloves, finely chopped
Coarse salt

1. Preheat the oven to 250°F.
2. Place the tomatoes cut-side up in a single layer on a baking sheet (you can line the pan with parchment paper).
3. Heat the oil in a small skillet. Add the garlic, and sauté 1 minute. Drizzle the oil and garlic over the tomatoes, and sprinkle lightly with the salt.
4. Place the tomatoes in the oven and bake for 2½ to 3 hours. The tomatoes should retain their shape. Let cool.

II. Melted Tomatoes

makes 24 pieces

Use summer tomatoes for this easy and velvety tomato recipe.

12 large, ripe red tomatoes
3 tablespoons extra-virgin olive oil
Sea salt
6 large garlic cloves, crushed

1. Preheat the oven to 250°F.
2. Bring a pot of water to a boil, add the tomatoes, and boil for 1 minute; drain and peel. Cut the tomatoes in half crosswise and seed. Put them on a foil-lined baking sheet, cut-side down. Drizzle with the oil. Sprinkle lightly with the sea salt. Sprinkle the crushed garlic over. Bake for 4 hours.

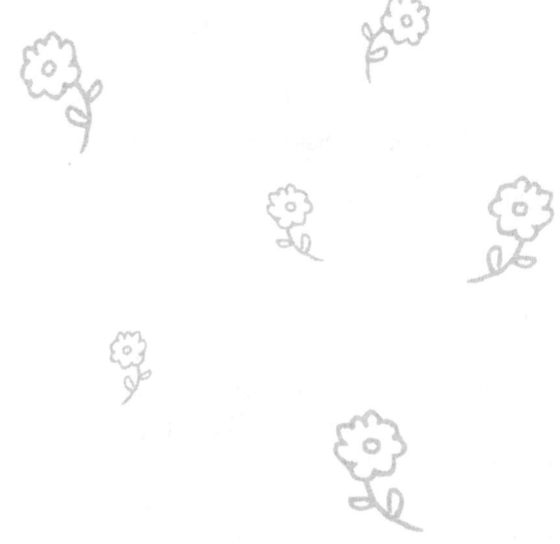

Grilled Vegetables (v)

Brendan Walsh
The Elms Restaurant and Tavern (Ridgefield, CT)

American food has a bright future in the hands of Brendan Walsh. Brendan is the owner and chef at The Elms Restaurant and Tavern in Ridgefield, Connecticut. He is passionate about taking fresh, seasonal, healthy ingredients and making even the simplest dish come alive with flavor.

makes 4 servings

When your parents pull out the grill, stick these vegetables on. They're a snap to cook, and they're just as good hot or cold. Use them to top pizza, put them on pasta, use them as a sandwich filling, or add them to a salad.

2 medium yellow or summer squash, both ends trimmed, sliced lengthwise into 1/2-inch-thick strips
2 medium zucchini, both ends trimmed, sliced lengthwise into 1/2-inch-thick strips
2 red bell peppers, sliced lengthwise into 1-inch-wide strips
1 medium eggplant, both ends trimmed, sliced crosswise into 1/2-inch-thick rounds
Extra-virgin olive oil
Salt and freshly milled black pepper

1. Preheat the grill.
2. Toss the prepared vegetables in a large bowl with enough oil to lightly coat them. Sprinkle with the salt and pepper, toss again, and let the vegetables marinate until the grill is medium-hot and the grill rack is hot.
3. Place the vegetables in a single layer on the grill rack over a medium-hot fire. When the vegetables are well marked, turn and grill the other side. The vegetables are finished cooking when they are tender and have nice dark grill marks on both sides. Remove from the heat. Serve warm or at room temperature.

Oven-Roasted Vegetables (v)

Brendan Walsh
The Elms Restaurant and Tavern (Ridgefield, CT)

makes 4 servings

When your parents won't pull out the grill, cook your vegetables in the oven instead. This is a recipe that works for lots of different vegetables, like carrots and asparagus and mushrooms. These vegetables are nice on pasta, pizza, rice, and bean salads and as a filling for a wrap with a little hummus or guacamole.

2 medium yellow or summer squash, both ends trimmed, sliced lengthwise into 1/4-inch-thick strips
2 medium zucchini, both ends trimmed, sliced lengthwise into 1/4-inch-thick strips
2 red bell peppers, sliced lengthwise into 1-inch-wide strips
1 medium eggplant, both ends trimmed, sliced crosswise into 1/4-inch-thick rounds
Extra-virgin olive oil
Salt and freshly milled black pepper

1. Preheat the oven to 425°F.
2. Toss the prepared vegetables in a large bowl with enough oil to lightly coat them. Sprinkle with the salt and pepper to taste, toss again, and let the vegetables marinate until the oven is hot.
3. Spread the vegetables out evenly on a large baking sheet. Roast 20 to 30 minutes, turning once or twice, until tender. Serve warm or at room temperature.

Russian Dressing (v)

Angelica Kitchen (New York City)

More of an icon than a restaurant, New York's Angelica Kitchen sets the standard that everyone else aspires to. From its sunny dining rooms, to its cheerful and professional service, to its inspired (vegan and organic) cuisine, to its reasonable prices, it's no wonder that Angelica doesn't just have customers, it practically has a fan club. This is a place that doesn't only believe in serving the community—it believes in giving back. All of the commitment and integrity of the people who run the place comes out in the dining experience. Oh yeah, the food tastes good, too!

makes 2 cups

While the Russian government is constantly changing, Russian dressing remains the same. This classic creamy dressing is best on sturdy lettuce, like iceberg and romaine. It's good as a sandwich spread and as a dip.

- 1/2 pound firm tofu
- 3 tablespoons rice syrup (see Note)
- 1 tablespoon fresh lemon juice
- 1 tablespoon canola oil
- 1 teaspoon prepared mustard
- 2/3 cup drained, finely chopped, oil-packed sun-dried tomatoes
- 2/3 cup minced pickles
- 1 tablespoon minced red onion
- 1/2 teaspoon salt

1. Combine the tofu, rice syrup, lemon juice, canola oil, and mustard in a food processor fitted with a steel blade. Puree until creamy.
2. Add the sun-dried tomatoes, pickles, onion, and salt. Pulse to combine. Refrigerate until ready to serve.

NOTE: Rice syrup is available in health food stores.

Basil-Curry Vinaigrette (v)

Jack Bishop
Cook's Illustrated magazine

Jack Bishop is one of those rare people who can write a cookbook that is as sensible and informative as the dishes are delicious. His recipes come out consistently great.

makes ½ cup

This bright, zesty dressing adds punch to any salad and is especially good on Asian greens like tatsoi and mizuma. Fresh basil is essential.

- 4 tablespoons olive oil
- 1½ tablespoons fresh lemon juice
- 1½ tablespoons white vinegar
- 1½ teaspoons honey
- ½ teaspoon curry powder
- Salt to taste
- 3 tablespoons minced fresh basil leaves

Whisk all the ingredients together, except the basil. Add the basil just before serving.

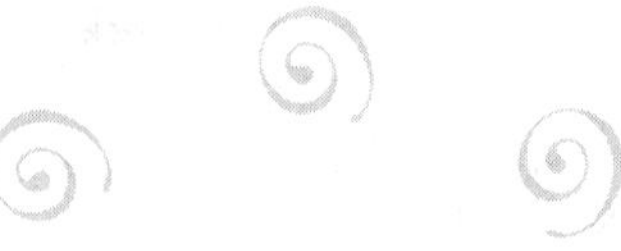

Cooked Chickpeas (v)

Jack Bishop
Cook's Illustrated magazine

This is a basic recipe for cooking chickpeas from scratch. You'll use these chickpeas for everything from hummus to soups. Best of all, you can do some of this in your sleep—soak the chickpeas overnight; then finish the rest of the preparation the next day.

- 2/3 cup dried chickpeas, soaked at least 8 hours, drained
- 2 garlic cloves, peeled
- 1 bay leaf
- 1 teaspoon salt

Bring 1 quart of water and the chickpeas, garlic, and bay leaf to a boil in a large saucepan; simmer until chickpeas are tender, about 45 minutes, adding the salt after 30 minutes of cooking. Drain, discard the garlic and bay leaf, and cool to room temperature.

Fruit Salsa (v)

Cary Neff
Miraval, Life in Balance Resort (Catalina, AZ)

makes about 4 cups

Aside from having the best name in the business (Chef Neff), Cary Neff knows how to make recipes that are a nice balance of healthy and yummy and simple. Here's a tropical salsa to brighten up sautéed tofu or a bowl of rice.

- 1/2 papaya, seeded and diced
- 1/2 pineapple, cored and diced
- 1/2 pint strawberries, hulled and diced
- 1 scallion, chopped
- 2 tablespoons honey
- 2 tablespoons fresh lime juice
- 1 tablespoon ground cumin
- 1 tablespoon fresh mint leaves, sliced into thin strips
- 1 tablespoon chopped cilantro

Combine all the ingredients, except the mint and cilantro, in a medium mixing bowl. Add the herbs just before serving.

Basil Mayonnaise

Brendan Walsh
The Elms Restaurant and Tavern (Ridgefield, CT)

makes about 2 cups

Jarred mayonnaise (Hellmann's is the best) can't begin to compare to this sublimely fresh taste. Two tips: Don't add the basil if you don't want to. Don't make it at all if you're freaked by E coli, since it calls for a raw egg.

- 1 large egg
- 1 tablespoon white wine vinegar
- 1 tablespoon Dijon mustard
- 2 teaspoons fresh lemon juice
- 1/2 teaspoon salt
- Pinch cayenne
- 1 cup canola-olive oil blend (1/2 c olive oil and 1/2 c canola)
- 1/4 cup minced fresh basil leaves

1. Combine the egg, vinegar, mustard, lemon juice, salt, and cayenne in a blender or food processor fitted with the steel blade; blend until the mixture is frothy, about 15 seconds.
2. With the machine running, add the oil in a thin, steady stream through the hole in the blender lid or the feed tube of the food processor. The egg mixture will transform itself into a smooth thick mayonnaise once all the oil has been added. Add the basil, and blend just until combined, about 3 seconds. Refrigerate until ready to use.

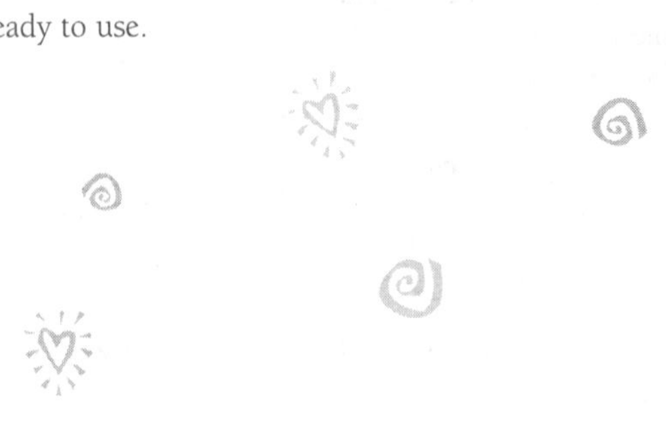

Focaccia (v)

Brendan Walsh
The Elms Restaurant and Tavern (Ridgefield, CT)

makes one 9- × 12-inch focaccia

Making focaccia from scratch is a labor of love; definitely a recipe to make with a friend. But once you get the hang of making your own focaccia, you will be hooked. P.S.: You can make this free form on a baking sheet. And speaking of love, how about a heart-shaped focaccia for Valentine's Day, topped with Ultra Tomatoes (p. 101)?

for the dough

One 1/4-ounce package active dry yeast, about 2 1/4 teaspoons
6 tablespoons extra-virgin olive oil
3 cups bread flour
1 teaspoon salt

for the topping:

1 small onion, halved and sliced thin
1 tablespoon fennel seeds, toasted
Sea salt

1. To make the dough, pour 1 cup warm water (110°F) into a 2-cup glass measuring cup and sprinkle in the yeast. Allow the yeast to soften and swell slightly, about 5 minutes. Stir in 2 tablespoons of the oil.
2. In the work bowl of a food processor fitted with a steel blade, pulse together the flour and salt. Continue to pulse while pouring in the liquid through the feed tube and until the mixture forms a ball. Process the dough until smooth and elastic, 30 to 40 seconds.
3. Transfer the dough to a large, lightly oiled bowl. Lightly oil a piece of plastic wrap large enough to cover the bowl. Cover the bowl tightly with the plastic wrap, oiled side down. Let the dough rise

in a warm area until doubled in size, 1 to 2 hours. Punch the dough down, recover tightly, and refrigerate 8 hours or overnight.

4. Oil a 9- × 12-inch metal baking pan with 2 tablespoons of the oil. Place the dough in the pan and, using your fingertips, gently press to fit evenly into the pan. If the dough is stubborn, let it rest about 15 minutes, covered with the plastic wrap; then try again. Let the dough rise again, covered, in a warm area until doubled in size, about 1 hour.
5. Preheat oven to 400°F.
6. Uncover and gently dimple the dough with your fingertips, being careful not to deflate the dough completely.
7. To top the dough, drizzle it with the remaining 2 tablespoons of oil. Sprinkle the onion, fennel seeds, and sea salt evenly over the top.
8. Bake 50 to 60 minutes, until the focaccia is golden brown and has a hollow sound when tapped in the center. Transfer to a wire rack to cool. When cool enough to handle, remove the focaccia from the pan. Serve warm.

VARIATIONS: Instead of onion and fennel seeds, try topping the focaccia with 1 tablespoon toasted sesame seeds and sea salt to taste. Or top with 1 cup of diced vegetables of your choice.

Basic Brown Rice

(V, if made without butter)

Jack Bishop
Cook's Illustrated magazine

makes 3 cups

If they can send a man to the moon, how come nobody can figure out how to make brown rice that doesn't come out sticky, gloppy, overcooked, and leaden? Finally, a recipe that gives you fluffy, chewy, tender, tasty brown rice every time.

Use long-, medium-, or short-grain rice in this recipe. If you own a rice cooker, follow the instructions, which call for less water, fat, and salt.

1 cup brown rice
2 teaspoons olive oil or butter
1 teaspoon salt

1. Bring 6 cups of water to a boil in a large pot. Stir in the rice, oil, and salt. Simmer briskly, uncovered, until the rice is almost tender, about 30 minutes.
2. Drain the rice into a steamer basket that fits inside the pot. Add about 1 inch of water to the bottom of the pot. Place the steamer basket in the pot; cover and steam until tender, 5 to 10 minutes. Scoop the rice into a bowl and fluff gently with a fork.

VARIATION: To cook in a rice cooker, stir 2¼ cups water, 1 cup brown rice, 1 teaspoon oil or butter, and ½ teaspoon salt in the cooking chamber. Cover and cook according to the manufacturer's directions. If rice ends up too crunchy for your taste, add several tablespoons of water and restart the machine. The rice cooker will shut off when the additional water has been absorbed.

Hummus (Chickpea Puree) (v)

Matthew Kenney
Matthew's (New York City)

He grew up in Maine and wound up being the authority on Mediterranean cuisine in New York. Go figure. And Matthew Kenney's not just a genius in the kitchen—he's practically an empire. Currently, he's got three successful restaurants in New York (a fourth is pending) and a best-selling cookbook.

Homemade hummus, toasted pita, black olives . . . Heaven! You can substitute canned chickpeas if you don't tell Matthew; then start at Step 2.

- 1 cup dried chickpeas, soaked at least 8 hours
- 1/4 cup tahini
- 2 garlic cloves, finely minced
- 1/4 cup fresh lemon juice
- Salt
- Cayenne

1. Drain the chickpeas and rinse well under running water. Place in a pot and add 4 cups of cold water. Bring the water to a boil over high heat; reduce the heat to medium-low, and cook until very soft, at least 45 minutes. Drain the chickpeas, reserving any liquid.
2. Transfer the chickpeas to a food processor fitted with the steel blade. Add the tahini, garlic, and lemon juice. Puree, adding the reserved cooking liquid or enough cold water to achieve a spreadable consistency. Season with salt and cayenne to taste. Serve at room temperature.

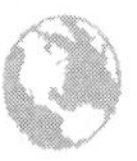

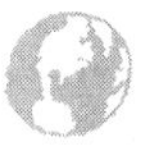

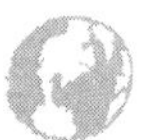

Salsa Verde (v)

Melissa Hamilton

makes about 1/2 cup

Not the kind of salsa you use as a dip, this refreshing emerald green sauce can be drizzled on everything from crusty bread to grilled vegetables to scrambled eggs or scrambled tofu.

- 2 tablespoons minced fresh parsley
- 2 tablespoons extra-virgin olive oil
- 1 tablespoon fresh lemon juice
- 1 tablespoon minced fresh basil leaves
- 1 tablespoon minced pitted green olives
- 1½ teaspoons minced drained capers
- 1 medium garlic clove, minced
- Salt and freshly milled black pepper to taste

Stir all the ingredients together in a small bowl. Serve at room temperature.

Pesto

Recipe courtesy of *Saveur* magazine

Basil's most glorious moment. This sunny green summer sauce gives plain pasta a reason to live. Pesto is also a wonderful way to top thick slices of summer tomatoes.

- 2 tablespoons pine nuts
- ½ teaspoon salt
- 2 garlic cloves, chopped
- 2 cups packed fresh basil leaves
- ½ cup extra-virgin olive oil
- 2 tablespoons grated Parmigiano-Reggiano cheese

Pulse the pine nuts and salt in a food processor fitted with the steel blade until finely ground. Add the garlic and basil, and drizzle in the olive oil. Add the cheese and process into a smooth paste.

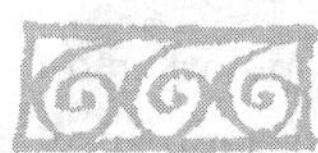

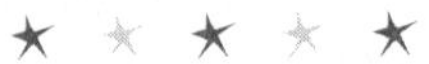

Miso Soup (v)

Angelica Kitchen (New York City)

makes 2 quarts

This traditional Asian soup is enriched with seaweed. It's a little labor intensive but so good you won't mind.

One 2-inch piece wakame (available at health food stores)
One 3-inch piece kombu (available at health food stores)
1 cup matchstick pieces carrot
1 cup thin half-circle slices onion
7 tablespoons barley miso or other miso
1 cup ½-inch cubes tofu
2 scallions, white and green parts sliced thin, for garnish

1. Soak the wakame in 2 cups of water. Set aside.
2. Add 4 cups water and the kombu to a medium saucepan. Bring to a simmer, and cook gently for 2 minutes. Remove the kombu, reserving it for another use (chopped into a stew or cooked with any grain or bean).
3. Strain the wakame soaking water into the saucepan. Add the carrot and onion. Chop the wakame into bite-sized pieces, and add to the saucepan. Bring the soup to a simmer, cover and cook gently over medium-low heat until the vegetables are tender, about 15 minutes.
4. Strain ½ cup of the soup stock into a small bowl; add the miso and stir to dissolve. Pour the miso mixture into the saucepan. Add the tofu and simmer 1 minute. Serve garnished with the scallions.

Lentil Soup (v)

Angelica Kitchen (New York City)

makes 2 quarts

Remember why we love dried lentils so much? Because we don't have to presoak or precook them! This is a nice, homey soup that sparkles with a hint of zesty lemon.

1 tablespoon extra-virgin olive oil
1 1/2 cups diced onions
Sea salt
1 cup diced carrots
1/2 cup diced celery, with leaves
1 garlic clove, crushed
1 bay leaf
2 teaspoons minced fresh herbs (such as sage, thyme, or rosemary), or 1 teaspoon dried
1 cup sorted and rinsed lentils
One 3-inch piece kombu
Juice of 1/2 lemon
Freshly milled black pepper
2 scallions, thinly sliced, for garnish

1. Warm the olive oil over medium heat in a heavy-bottomed soup pot. Add onions and a pinch of salt, cook 8 to 10 minutes, stirring occasionally. Add the carrots, celery, garlic, bay leaf, and herbs; sauté 5 minutes. Add the lentils, kombu, and 6 cups water; bring to a boil. Lower the heat to medium-low; cover and simmer until the lentils are tender, 40 to 50 minutes.
2. Remove and discard the kombu. Stir in the lemon juice; add salt and pepper to taste. Simmer for 3 minutes. Serve garnished with the scallions.

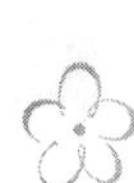
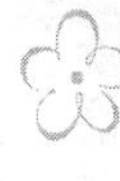
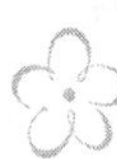
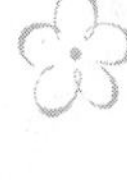
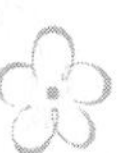
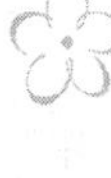
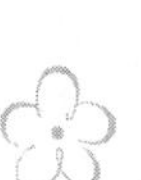
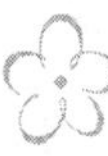

Pasta and White Bean Soup with Garlic and Rosemary (v)

Jack Bishop
The Complete Italian Vegetarian Cookbook
(Houghton Mifflin, 1997)

makes 6 servings

This classic pasta and bean soup, called pasta e fagioli, *is found all over Italy. You can use two 19-ounce cans of cannellini beans, drained and rinsed, if you don't want to cook the beans yourself.*

- 1/4 cup extra-virgin olive oil plus more for drizzling over the soup
- 4 large garlic cloves, minced
- 2 teaspoons minced fresh rosemary leaves
- 1 1/2 cups drained canned whole tomatoes, chopped
- Salt and freshly milled black pepper
- 7 cups vegetable stock or water
- 6 ounces small pasta, such as small elbows or shells
- 4 cups cooked cannellini beans

1. Heat the oil in a large soup kettle or stockpot. Add the garlic and rosemary, and sauté over medium heat for about 2 minutes.
2. Add the tomatoes and a generous amount of salt and pepper. Simmer until the tomatoes soften, 3 to 4 minutes.
3. Add the stock, and bring to a boil. Lower the heat and simmer 5 minutes. Add the pasta to the simmering broth and cook until almost tender, 7 to 10 minutes.
4. Add the beans, and simmer 2 to 3 minutes to blend the flavors and finish cooking the pasta. Adjust the seasonings. Serve immediately with a drizzle of oil to taste.

Minestrone

(V, if you don't add cheese)

Recipe courtesy of *Saveur* magazine

makes 4 servings

This Italian vegetable soup is made heartier with the addition of beans and pasta. Cauliflower, turnips, and carrots may be used in place of or in addition to the vegetables called for. Top with fresh pesto, if you want to add another layer of flavor.

1 ounce dried porcini mushrooms
1/4 pound Swiss chard
1/4 pound spinach
Salt
2 small zucchini, diced
2 medium white potatoes, peeled and diced
2 Japanese eggplants, peeled and diced
2 tablespoons extra-virgin olive oil
2 cups dry tubetti pasta
2 cups cooked white beans
2 tablespoons homemade Pesto (page 113), or store-bought
Freshly milled black pepper

1. Soak the mushrooms in 2 cups of warm water until soft, about 20 minutes. Remove the mushrooms, rinse, chop, and set aside. Pour the mushroom water through a coffee filter and reserve. Wash the chard and spinach in several changes of cold water. Trim and discard the stalks from the chard and the stems from the spinach. Chop the leaves.
2. Bring the mushroom water and 6 cups salted water to a boil in a large pot. Add the mushrooms, chard, spinach, zucchinis, potatoes, eggplants, and olive oil. Reduce the heat to low, and simmer, uncovered, for 1 hour.

3. Add the pasta to soup; cook about 10 minutes. Add the beans, and cook 5 minutes longer. Stir in the pesto, and season with salt and pepper. Serve hot or, in the Genovese tradition, at room temperature. If desired, sprinkle with grated Parmigiano-Reggiano cheese.

Mushroom Barley Soup (v)

Angelica Kitchen (New York City)

makes 2 quarts

It's the middle of February, it's 20° below, it's been snowing for three days straight. Brrrr. . . . If you want something to warm your soul, this is your soup.

- 1/2 cup pearl barley
- 1 tablespoon extra-virgin olive oil
- 2 cups thinly sliced mushrooms
- 1 cup diced onion
- 1/2 cup chopped carrots
- 1/2 cup chopped celery
- 1/2 cup chopped green cabbage
- 1 garlic clove, minced
- 1 teaspoon sea salt
- 2 tablespoons minced fresh dill
- 2 tablespoons shoyu or tamari

1. Rinse the barley, drain, and combine with 6 cups of water in a heavy soup pot; bring to boil over high heat. Reduce the heat to medium-low; simmer, covered, until the barley is tender, 45 minutes.
2. Meanwhile, heat the olive oil in a heavy-bottomed skillet or saucepan over medium heat. Add the mushrooms, onion, carrot, celery, cabbage, garlic, and salt; sauté 3 to 5 minutes. Reduce the

heat to medium-low, cover, and sweat the vegetables until tender, about 15 minutes. Remove from the heat.

3. When the barley is tender, stir in the cooked vegetables, dill, and shoyu; simmer 10 minutes. Serve hot.

Wood-Grilled Vegetable Sandwich on Focaccia

Brendan Walsh
The Elms Restaurant and Tavern (Ridgefield, CT)

makes 1 sandwich

At his restaurant, Brendan likes to grill the vegetables over a wood fire and then melt the cheese on top in a warm oven before putting the whole thing together. You don't need to melt the cheese if you don't feel like it. Also, Oven-Roasted Vegetables (page 104) work as well as the grilled ones.

- 1 slice homemade Focaccia (page 109) or store-bought
- 2 teaspoons Basil Mayonnaise (page 108) or store-bought mayonnaise mixed with teaspoon fresh basil to taste
- 2 leaves red lettuce
- 1 serving Grilled Vegetables (page 103), preferably warm
- 1/4 cup Italian fontina cheese, grated to taste
- Salt and freshly milled pepper
- 1/2 ripe tomato, sliced

1. Slice the Focaccia in half lengthwise. Spread each half with some Basil Mayonnaise.
2. Place a leaf of the lettuce on one half, and arrange some grilled vegetables on top. Sprinkle with the cheese. Season to taste with the salt and pepper.
3. Cover with tomato slices and the other lettuce leaf. Top with the other half of the Focaccia.

Make-a-Hamburger-Jealous Burger (v)

John Gottfried
Gourmet Garage (New York City)

John's Gourmet Garage in New York City offers the most incredible selection of local and exotic fruits and vegetables. A former food editor and critic, John not only selects the best produce but knows just what to do with it when he gets it home and starts cooking.

makes 4 sandwiches

John believes that when it comes to burgers, it's not about meat or no meat, it's really about how juicy and moist the burgers are. Here's a scrumptious mushroom burger that proves his point.

- 4 kaiser or hard rolls
- 1/4 cup olive oil
- 1 1/2 pounds large button mushrooms, wiped clean with damp cloth or paper towel
- 1 tablespoon fresh thyme leaves or 1/2 teaspoon dried
- 1 medium garlic clove, minced
- Juice of 1/4 lemon
- Salt and freshly milled black pepper
- 4 crisp lettuce leaves

1. Preheat the broiler.
2. Slice the kaiser rolls in half and hollow them out; save the bread crumbs for another use. Brush the inside of the rolls with a little of the oil and broil, oiled side up, until lightly toasted. Set aside.
3. Remove the stems from mushroom caps; coarsely chop the stems. Heat the remaining oil in a large skillet over medium-high heat and add the caps. Cover and cook, turning once, until heated through, about 5 minutes. Add the chopped stems, thyme, and garlic. Continue to simmer, uncovered, stirring occasionally, until heated

through, about 2 minutes. Squeeze the lemon juice over the mixture. Season to taste with the salt and pepper.

4. Divide the cooked mushroom caps among the four roll bottoms with the underside of the mushroom cap facing up. Fill the mushroom caps with the mushroom stem mixture. Add a lettuce leaf, and cover with a roll top. Serve warm.

Juicy Portobello Burger

(V, if made without the mayo)

John Gottfried
Gourmet Garage (New York City)

makes 4 sandwiches

How good is this mushroom burger? So good, John swears, that just one juicy bite will convert even the most die-hard hamburger fan.

- 4 kaiser or hard rolls
- 4 large portobello mushrooms, stemmed
- 6 tablespoons extra-virgin olive oil
- 2 tablespoons fresh thyme or chopped rosemary leaves
- 2 garlic cloves, minced very fine
- 1 small lemon
- Salt and freshly milled black pepper
- 1 large, ripe tomato, sliced (optional)
- Mayonnaise (optional)

1. Preheat the broiler.
2. Slice the kaiser rolls in half and hollow out; save the bread crumbs for another use. Brush the inside of the rolls with a little oil and broil, oiled side up, until lightly toasted. Set aside.
3. For best results, although this isn't necessary, trim away most of the dark gills on the underside of each mushroom cap. Brush the

trimmed sides generously with olive oil, and sprinkle with the thyme and garlic.

4. Place the caps, trimmed side up under the broiler for about 3 minutes; turn the caps over and broil for another 2 minutes. Since broilers vary, keep your eye on the mushrooms. Remove the caps from broiler, turn gill side up, and season with a small squeeze of lemon juice and the salt and pepper to taste.
5. Place each cap on a roll bottom. Top with the tomato slices and mayonnaise, if desired. Cover with the roll top. Serve warm.

Grilled Vegetable Flatbread Sandwich with Hummus (v)

Matthew Kenney
Matthew's (New York City)

makes 1 sandwich

Another take on a grilled-vegetable sandwich. Matthew sells this to go at Mezze, his New York bistro, and it is a huge favorite with the ravenous lunch crowd.

- 1 small zucchini, trimmed and cut lengthwise into 1/4-inch strips
- 1 small eggplant, trimmed and cut lengthwise into 1/4-inch strips
- 1 small red pepper, cut into 1-inch strips
- 4 tablespoons extra-virgin olive oil
- Salt and freshly milled black pepper
- 1/2 cup fresh greens (arugula, mesclun, or lettuce of your choice)

2 teaspoons fresh lemon juice
1 slice flatbread
2 tablespoons homemade Hummus (page 112) or store-bought

1. Preheat the grill.
2. Toss the prepared vegetables with 2 tablespoons of the oil and salt and pepper to taste. Set aside until grill is medium-hot and the grill grate is hot.
3. Toss the greens with remaining 2 tablespoons of the oil, the lemon juice, and salt and pepper to taste.
4. Grill the vegetables until the flesh is marked and begins to soften. Remove from the grill and set aside.
5. Smooth the hummus onto center of the flatbread. Arrange the greens in the center, in a horizontal column. Place the grilled vegetables on top of the greens. Roll the sandwich tightly, cut on an angle, and serve immediately.

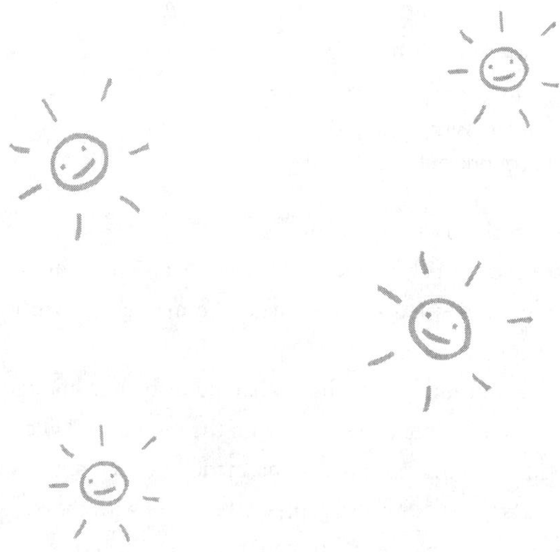

Tempeh Reuben Sandwich (v)

Angelica Kitchen (New York City)

makes 4 sandwiches

Delectable Eastern European dish meets hip health-conscious downtown vegan. Result: love at first bite. Here's the Reuben, as interpreted by Angelica's creative guru, chef Peter Berley.

1 pound tempeh, cut into sandwich-size pieces and sliced in half horizontally

for the marinade

- 1 1/3 cups apple cider or apple juice
- 3 tablespoons shoyu
- 3 tablespoons prepared mustard, preferably grainy
- 1 teaspoon ground cumin
- 1 teaspoon ground caraway seed
- 1 garlic clove, minced
- Pinch cayenne
- 1/3 cup canola oil

for the sandwich

- 8 slices bread, seeded rye or your choice
- Russian Dressing (page 105)
- White sauerkraut

1. Preheat the oven to 350°F.
2. Place the tempeh in a steamer, and steam 5 to 7 minutes.
3. While tempeh is steaming, make the marinade. Whisk all the ingredients together.
4. Transfer steamed tempeh to a baking dish large enough to hold it in a single layer. Barely cover with the marinade. Bake, uncovered, about 35 minutes, until the marinade has been absorbed.
5. To make the sandwiches, spread the bread with the Russian Dressing. Layer four slices with the tempeh and sauerkraut. Cover with the remaining bread. Serve warm.

Pan-Roasted Tofu with Green Bean Salad (v)

Larry Forgione
An American Place (New York City)

Back when most American cooks were heating up frozen green beans, Larry Forgione was preaching the virtues of fresh, seasonal food and American ingredients. Then he actually tracked the native foods down: he had foragers searching for wild salad greens and mushrooms in fields on Long Island. If it is possible for a chef to have the equivalent of music's perfect pitch, Larry does. He makes his ingredients harmonize and his dishes sing.

makes 4 servings

This makes a really impressive presentation—a great marriage of tastes and textures. It looks like endless work, but it's really just endless ingredients.

3 ounces favorite steak sauce
1 ounce tamari
1/2 ounce rice wine vinegar
1/4 teaspoon chili oil
1 teaspoon toasted sesame oil
Salt and freshly ground black pepper
1 piece extra-firm organic tofu, drained and sliced into 4 thick slices
1/2 pound trimmed green beans, cooked al dente and chilled
1/2 red bell pepper, stemmed, seeded, and cut into thin strips
1 cup cooked black beans, rinsed
1/2 teaspoon minced garlic
1 tablespoon black sesame seeds (optional)
1 tablespoon chopped fresh cilantro
1 tablespoon olive oil

1. In a small bowl, prepare the dressing by whisking together the steak sauce, tamari, rice vinegar, chili oil, and sesame oil. Season to taste with salt and pepper.
2. Spoon 2 tablespoons of the dressing onto a plate. Place the tofu on top, and spoon 1 tablespoon of the dressing over each slice. Cover and refrigerate 1 to 2 hours.
3. Finish the salad by tossing the green beans, bell pepper, black beans, garlic, sesame seeds, and cilantro with a few tablespoons of the dressing in a medium-size bowl. Divide vegetables among four plates.
4. In a heavy nonstick sauté pan, heat the olive oil over high heat until quite hot. Carefully lift each piece of tofu from the marinade and add it to the pan; cook for 1 minute. Flip each piece over and cook 1 minute more. Place one piece of tofu on each plate. Add any remaining dressing to the sauté pan, heat briefly, then spoon over the salad. Serve immediately.

Brown Rice and Chickpea Salad with Basil-Curry Vinaigrette (v)

Jack Bishop

makes 4 servings for a light main course

Brown rice with lots and lots of pizazz. And this isn't just a recipe . . . it's a guide for making all sorts of rice salads: Combine 3 cups of cooked brown rice with a mixture of 3 cups of cooked vegetables or cooked beans. Add 1/4 to 1/2 cup of toasted nuts for crunch. Then toss and mix with any vinaigrette.

- 1 recipe Cooked Chickpeas (page 106)
- 3 cups Basic Brown Rice (page 110), preferably medium-grain or basmati, cooled to room temperature
- 1 large red bell pepper, diced small
- 1/4 cup lightly toasted sliced almonds
- 1 recipe Basil-Curry Vinaigrette (page 106)

Mix the chickpeas, rice, bell pepper, and almonds in a medium bowl. Pour the dressing over, and toss to combine. Can be refrigerated for up to 4 hours.

Easy Summer Potato Salad (v)

David Page
Home (New York City)

What would you expect from a man from Wisconsin whose restaurant is called Home? Nothing less than all-American food that is down-to-earth, unpretentious, and well . . . homey. Nothing fancy in David's cooking—just his sense of how satisfying a simple dish can be. POP QUIZ: *Guess what David named the take-out place around the corner from his restaurant? Give up? Home Away From Home!*

makes 6 servings

It doesn't get any easier or better than this. The key to success here is to slice the potatoes when they're warm and immediately toss them with the oil and vinegar so they really absorb the flavors.

- 3 pounds small white potatoes, or Yukon gold potatoes
- 1 medium bunch scallions, minced
- 1 1/2 cups olive oil
- 3/4 cup apple cider vinegar
- Salt and freshly milled black pepper

1. In a medium pot, cover the potatoes with cold, salted water and bring to a boil over medium-high heat. Reduce the heat and simmer until just tender. Drain.
2. While the potatoes are still warm, slice them directly into a mixing bowl. Toss with the scallions, olive oil, vinegar, and salt and pepper to taste.

Three-Grain Salad with Cucumber and Tomato (v)

David Page
Home (New York City)

makes 6 servings

This refreshing salad is one-step plus prep. Red rice is a Native American rice. You're likely to find it under the name Wehani rice at a health food or gourmet store. It has a pleasant nutty flavor and resilient texture.

- 1 1/2 cups cooked red rice, cooled
- 1 1/2 cups cooked barley, cooled
- 1 1/2 cups cooked cracked wheat, cooled
- 1 English cucumber, seeded, peeled, and cut into small dice
- 1 cup diced tomato
- 1/2 cup chopped parsley
- 3/4 cup olive oil
- 1/4 cup fresh lemon juice
- Salt and pepper

Combine all the ingredients; toss. Serve slightly chilled or at room temperature.

Internet Smoothie (v)

Nadine R. Ames
(Ithaca, New York)

When this recipe came beaming in from cyberspace to Phoebe's computer, it made us laugh (vegetarians need to laugh). Thanks, Nadine!

Date: Mon, 13 Apr 94 10:00.14 EDT 1 frozen banana (peel a very ripe/nearly overripe banana and put in freezer, naked) 1 cup (approx.) your favorite fruit + I like strawberries! 1/2 cup to 1 cup apple juice or nonfat soy milk (or whatever, you get the idea, amount depends on how thick or thin you like) Blenderize.

Tropical Fruit Smoothie (v)

Joan Huey
Blanche's Organic Café (New York City)

Organic, free-range, farm-raised, dairy-free, guilt-free—everything about Blanche's is p.c. and prepared with loving care. A hip, healthy restaurant with a lot of soul. And how can you not love a place that sells a whey-protein fruit shake called Whey To Go.

Thanks for recipe help to former Blanche's chefs Christopher Gaddess of New York City and Alexis Bondaroff (now at Organica in Brooklyn).

This is a great shake for breakfast, or any time of day. Some tips from the folks at Blanche's: "For best results, always use ripe fruit. Some fruits are hard to find or too expensive during the winter, so try dicing up the fruit while it's in season and store in a zipper-locking bag in the freezer." The bee pollen is for energy!

1 cup diced fruit, use any combo of mango, papaya, or pineapple
1 ripe banana
1 cup fresh orange juice
1 cup ice
1 teaspoon bee pollen (optional)

Place all the ingredients in a blender; blend until smooth.

Phoebe's Warm White Bean Puree (v)

Stephanie Pierson and Phoebe Connell
(South Salem, New York)

makes about 4 cups

Chances are, you'll make this so much that it will soon be your own. Then you can give it your name. Phoebe loves this on toasted slices of French bread. Try not to use dried rosemary; it doesn't work anywhere near as well as fresh, and since just about every supermarket (even in January in Nebraska) sells fresh rosemary, you can probably find it.

1 medium garlic clove, minced
3 tablespoons extra-virgin olive oil or more to taste

- ½ teaspoon chopped fresh rosemary leaves
- 4 cups cooked cannellini beans or two 19-ounce cans, drained and rinsed
- Salt and pepper

1. In a medium skillet or saucepan, bring ¼ cup water, the garlic, olive oil, and rosemary to a simmer over medium heat. Simmer 1 minute. Stir in the beans. Continue to cook, stirring frequently, until the bean mixture is heated through. Remove from the heat.
2. Mash the warm beans into a chunky puree with the tines of a fork or pulse in a food processor until coarsely pureed.
3. Transfer the puree to a bowl. Season with salt and pepper to taste.

Sandbox Toasted Granola

John Holm
Sandbox (New York City)

makes about 3 pounds

Everything's fresh and enticing at Sandbox, a spiffy New York take-out place. But their granola is truly addictive. John Holm was kind enough to share his recipe. Actually, he gave us a store recipe, which would make forty-six pounds and serve about 150 people. We cut it down a bit.

- ¾ cup honey
- 4 ounces unsalted butter
- ½ cup packed brown sugar
- 5½ cups rolled oats
- 1½ cups shredded, sweetened coconut
- ½ cup sunflower seeds
- ½ cup pumpkin seeds
- ½ cup walnut pieces

$^{1}/_{2}$ cup slivered almonds
$^{1}/_{4}$ cup shelled, unsalted pistachio nuts

1. Preheat the oven to 325°F.
2. In a medium saucepan, combine the honey, butter, and brown sugar; heat over low heat until the butter melts.
3. Meanwhile, in a large mixing bowl, combine the remaining ingredients. Add the warmed honey mixture. Stir well to combine.
4. Working in batches, if necessary, spread mixture out evenly on baking sheet.
5. Bake until golden brown, stirring periodically to ensure an even coloration. Let cool completely before storing in airtight container, about 30 minutes.

So one day in April, Tom (my husband) and I are giving Phoebe a ride to school, and Phoebe (not having had time for breakfast) is in the backseat eating Sandbox Toasted Granola. Suddenly she lets out a high-pitched scream and shouts hysterically, "Pull over! Now!" Tom and I whip around to see what in the world could have happened to her. A bee? An alien? Worse! It turns out that a piece of granola has managed to dislodge her pierced tongue ring. Just to let you know that it isn't just tasty, it's really crunchy.

Stovetop Macaroni and Cheese

Pam Anderson
The Perfect Recipe (Houghton Mifflin, 1998)

Who could make better all-American meals than someone who is a lifelong cook, a food writer, and a mother of teenagers? Pam Anderson puts together recipes that let you have great home-cooked stuff without being a kitchen slave.

makes 4 main course servings or 6 to 8 side dish servings

The only macaroni and cheese recipe you'll ever need. Foolproof and fast. If you're in a major hurry, skip the bread crumb step.

- 1 cup fresh bread crumbs from French or Italian bread
- 2 teaspoons plus pinch salt
- 1 1/2 tablespoons unsalted butter, melted
- 2 large eggs
- One 12-ounce can evaporated milk
- 1/4 teaspoon hot red pepper sauce
- 2 teaspoons salt
- 1/4 teaspoon freshly milled black pepper
- 1 teaspoon dry mustard, dissolved in 1 teaspoon water
- 1/2 pound elbow macaroni
- 4 tablespoons unsalted butter
- 10 ounces sharp Wisconsin Cheddar, American, or Monterey Jack cheese, grated (about 3 cups)

1. Heat the oven to 350°F.
2. Mix the bread crumbs, pinch of salt, and melted butter together in a small baking pan. Bake 15 to 20 minutes, until golden brown and crisp; set aside.
3. Meanwhile, mix the eggs, 1 cup of the evaporated milk, the red pepper sauce, ½ teaspoon of the salt, the pepper, and mustard mixture in small bowl; set aside.
4. Heat 2 quarts of water to boil in large heavy-bottomed saucepan or Dutch oven. Add the remaining 1½ teaspoons of the salt and the macaroni; cook until almost tender, but still a little firm to the bite. Drain and return to the pan over medium heat. Add the 4 tablespoons of butter; toss to melt.
5. Pour the egg mixture over the macaroni along with three-quarters of the cheese; stir until thoroughly combined and the cheese starts to melt. Gradually add the remaining milk and cheese, stirring constantly, until the mixture is hot and creamy, about 5 minutes. Serve immediately, topped with the toasted bread crumbs.

Maple Baked Beans (v)

Ken Haedrich

Feeding the Healthy Vegetarian Family (Bantam, 1998)

makes 6 to 8 servings

So hearty and mellow, even the meat-eaters in your life will be hoping you've made enough for seconds. This cooks for hours and hours so it is not for the impatient or starving.

1 pound dried Great Northern beans
1/4 cup flavorless vegetable or safflower oil
1 cup chopped onion
1 green bell pepper, finely chopped
1 celery rib, finely chopped
2 garlic cloves, minced
1/2 cup canned tomato puree
1/2 cup maple syrup
3 tablespoons apple cider vinegar
2 tablespoons blackstrap molasses
2 tablespoons Dijon mustard
1 1/4 teaspoons salt
1 bay leaf
1/4 cup chopped fresh parsley
Freshly ground pepper

1. Pick over the beans, and rinse well. Put them in a large pot, and cover with about 3 inches water. Bring to a boil, cook uncovered for 2 minutes. Remove from the heat, cover, let stand for 1 hour; then drain.
2. Cover the beans generously with fresh water and bring to a boil. Gently boil, partially covered, until tender but not mushy, 1 to 1½ hours. Make sure they are tender, because the acidity of the liquid they'll bake in will prevent the beans from getting any softer. Drain, reserving the cooking water.
3. While the beans cook, heat the oil in a large skillet. Add the onion, pepper, and celery; sauté over medium-high heat about 6 minutes. Stir in the garlic; sauté 15 seconds more; then remove from the heat.
4. Preheat the oven to 325°F.
5. In a medium bowl, whisk together the remaining ingredients, adding 1½ cups of the bean cooking water. Transfer the beans, sautéed vegetables, and tomato mixture to a Dutch oven and stir gently to blend. Cover and bake 2 to 3 hours. Check the progress of the beans every hour, stirring them and checking the level of the liquid; if it gets too low, stir in a bit more bean water. When beans are done, the liquid should be fairly thick and saucy. Serve hot.

Classic Grilled Cheese Sandwiches

Melissa Hamilton

makes 2 sandwiches

Even if nothing in your life is perfect, you'll be happy to know your grilled cheese sandwich can be. There are endless additions to this perfection, but the extras are best sandwiched between the cheese. Try a few slices of ripe, in-season tomato or two or three tablespoons of caramelized onion.

- 3 ounces cheese (preferably mild Cheddar) or combination of cheeses, grated on the large holes of a box grater (about 1 cup, lightly packed)
- 4 slices ($^1/_2$ inch thick) firm white sandwich bread
- 2 tablespoons butter, melted

1. Heat a heavy 12-inch skillet over medium-low heat.
2. Meanwhile, sprinkle the cheese over two bread slices. Top each with a remaining bread slice, pressing down lightly to set.
3. Brush the sandwich tops completely with half the melted butter; place each sandwich, buttered side down, in the skillet. Brush the remaining side of each sandwich completely with the remaining butter. Cook until crisp and deep golden brown, 5 to 10 minutes per side, flipping the sandwiches back to the first side to reheat and crisp, about 15 seconds. Serve immediately.

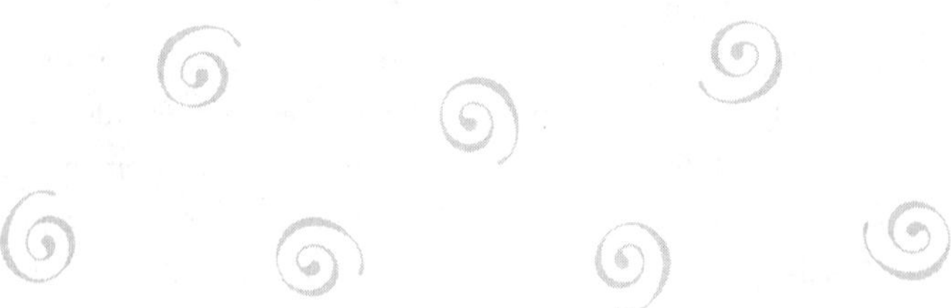

Pancakes and Cornbread

Brendan Walsh
The Elms Restaurant and Tavern (Ridgefield, CT)

makes about 14 pancakes or one 9-inch square cornbread

Here's one recipe that's really two-two-two recipes in one. You can use it to make either pancakes or cornbread just by adjusting the wet ingredients.

dry ingredients

- 1 cup all-purpose flour
- 1 cup cornmeal
- 1½ tablespoons sugar
- 3¾ teaspoons baking powder
- ½ teaspoon salt

wet ingredients

- 1 to 1½ cups milk
- 1½ to 2 tablespoons vegetable oil or unsalted butter, melted
- 1 to 2 large eggs, lightly beaten

Pancakes

1. Combine the dry mix ingredients. In a 2-cup glass measuring cup combine 1½ cups of milk, 1½ tablespoons of oil, and 1 egg. Whisk the wet ingredients into the dry mix to form a smooth batter.
2. Heat a very lightly oiled griddle or nonstick skillet over medium-high heat. For each pancake, pour approximately 3 tablespoons batter onto the hot surface. When bubbles form over the entire surface and the pancakes are golden underneath, quickly and carefully flip them, cook until the second side is golden and the pancakes are cooked through. Serve warm.

Can You Top This?

Here are Brendan's pancake topping suggestions:

Fresh fruit with a dollop of yogurt and a sprinkle of wheat germ.

Toss pineapple and banana slices with some sugar, sauté briefly; transfer to a bowl, stir in some vanilla, and serve over the warm pancakes.

Sautéed apples with cinnamon and brown sugar.

Sliced ripe pears with some chopped candied ginger.

A dollop of yogurt, crème fraîche, or sour cream with a plop of jam or jelly.

Cornbread

1. Preheat the oven to 350°F. Lightly coat a 9- × 9-inch baking pan with vegetable oil spray.
2. In a medium mixing bowl, combine the dry ingredients. In a 2-cup glass measuring cup combine 1 cup of milk, 2 tablespoons of oil, and 2 eggs. Whisk the wet ingredients into the dry mix to form a smooth, thick batter. Pour into the prepared pan. Bake 25 to 35 minutes, until golden brown and a toothpick inserted in center comes out clean.
3. Transfer to cooling rack. Best served warm.

Pizza Dough (v)

Pam Anderson
The Perfect Recipe (Houghton Mifflin, 1998)

makes 2 large, 4 medium, or 8 individual crusts

Maybe in Italy they don't think pizza is so all-American, but we know better. Make it from scratch (the food processor makes it less of a pain), and make the crust as thin or thick as you like.

- 1 envelope active dry yeast (2¼ teaspoons)
- 2 tablespoons olive oil
- 4 cups plus extra bread flour
- 1½ teaspoons salt
- Vegetable oil or spray for oiling the bowl

1. Pour ½ cup warm water (105°F) into 2-cup measuring cup. Sprinkle in the yeast; let stand until the yeast dissolves and swells, about 5 minutes. Add 1¼ cups of room-temperature water and the oil; stir to combine.
2. Pulse together the flour and salt in a food processor fitted with the steel blade. Continue pulsing while pouring the liquid ingredients (holding back a few tablespoons) through the feed tube. If the dough does not readily form into a ball, add the remaining liquid, and continue to pulse until a ball forms. Process until the dough is smooth and satiny, about 30 seconds longer.
3. The dough will be a bit tacky, so use a rubber spatula to turn it out onto lightly floured work surface; knead by hand with a few strokes to form smooth, round ball. Put the dough into deep, medium-large, oiled bowl; cover with a damp cloth. Let rise until doubled, about 2 hours.

Quick Tomato Sauce for Pizza (V)

Pam Anderson
The Perfect Recipe (Houghton Mifflin, 1998)

makes 3 cups

If you don't have time to cook this sauce or you're really lazy, simply mix the ingredients together, and set aside at room temperature for up to several hours. The heat from the oven will "cook" the sauce while the thin-crust pizza is baking.

2 large garlic cloves, minced
2 tablespoons extra-virgin olive oil
One 28-ounce can crushed tomatoes
Salt and ground black pepper

Heat the garlic with the oil in saucepan over medium heat. When the garlic starts to sizzle, add the tomatoes. Simmer, uncovered, until the sauce is thick enough to mound on the spoon, about 15 minutes. Season to taste with the salt and pepper.

Homemade Plain Cheese Pizza

Pam Anderson
The Perfect Recipe (Houghton Mifflin, 1998)

Making your own pizza is one of life's highest achievements. The only problem is that from now on most other pizzas will suffer by comparison. NOTE: *Buy a pizza stone at a housewares store—it really improves the crust.*

1 recipe Pizza Dough (page 139)
Flour for dusting hands and work surface

Semolina flour or cornmeal for dusting peel
Extra-virgin olive oil for brushing on dough
1 1/2 cups Quick Tomato Sauce for Pizza (page 140)
4 ounces mozzarella cheese, shredded (1 cup)
1/4 cup grated Parmesan cheese

1. Place a pizza stone in the oven, and preheat to 425°F (this will take at least 30 minutes).
2. Meanwhile, turn the prepared dough out onto lightly floured work surface, and use chef's knife or dough scraper to cut the dough into halves, quarters, or eighths, depending on number and size of pizzas desired. Form each piece into ball and cover loosely with a damp cloth. Let the dough relax at least 5 minutes but no more than 30 minutes.
3. Working with one piece of dough at a time and keeping others covered, flatten the ball into a disk using the palms of your hand. Starting at the center and working outward, use your fingertips to press the dough out to about 1/2 inch thick. Use one hand to hold the dough in place and other hand to stretch the dough outward; rotate the dough one-quarter turn, and stretch again. Repeat turning and stretching until the dough will not stretch any farther. Let relax 5 minutes; continue stretching until it reaches the correct diameter. The dough should be about 1/4 inch thick. (For large pizzas, let the dough relax another 5 minutes and stretch again.) Use your palm to flatten the edge of the dough. Transfer to a pizza peel that has been lightly coated with semolina flour.
4. Brush the dough round very lightly with the olive oil. Prick all over with a fork. Spread on a portion of the tomato sauce, leaving a 1/2-inch border around the edges uncovered. Using a quick jerking action, immediately slide the dough off the peel and onto the heated pizza stone. Bake 3 to 10 minutes, until the edges start to brown. Remove from the oven. Sprinkle with a portion of the cheeses. Return to the oven and continue baking 2 to 3 minutes more, until the cheeses are completely melted. Remove from the oven, slice into wedges, and serve immediately.

Asian Corn Fritters

Jerry Weinberg
Five Spice Café (Burlington, VT)

makes twenty to thirty 2½-inch fritters

I asked my neighbor Kate what she particularly liked about going to the University of Vermont, and she said, "The Five Spice Café." For vegetarians and non, the café's mouthwatering curry corn fritters are great.

for the fritters

One 15-ounce can creamed corn
3/4 cup all-purpose flour
1/2 tablespoon baking powder (nonaluminum)
1/2 tablespoon brown sugar or maple syrup
3 large eggs, lightly beaten
1/2 tablespoon yellow Indian curry
Grated zest of 1/2 lemon
1/4 teaspoon white pepper
1 1/2 tablespoons minced garlic
1 1/2 tablespoons light soy
1/2 tablespoon grated ginger
7 ounces canned whole-kernel corn, drained
Oil for cooking

for the dipping sauce

1/2 cup hoisin sauce
1 tablespoon Asian sesame oil
1 teaspoon grated orange zest, preferably organic

1. To make the fritters, blend all the fritter ingredients, except the whole-kernel corn and oil, very thoroughly. Stir in the whole-kernel corn, and mix well.
2. In large sauté pan heat 2 tablespoons oil (preferably extra-virgin olive oil) on medium-high heat. Spoon in 2 to 3 tablespoons of the batter for each 2½-inch fritter. When bubbles form through much of the fritter, carefully turn with a spatula. Reduce the heat if the fritters are much darker than golden. Drain on paper towels and keep warm in a low oven. Add more oil as needed, but not too much. Continue frying the fritters.
3. To make the dipping sauce combine all the sauce ingredients in a small bowl. Serve with the warm fritters.

Golden Tofu (v)

Deborah Madison

Vegetarian Cooking for Everyone (Broadway Books, 1997)

If anyone in America can convert the hamburger and meatloaf crowd, it's Deborah Madison. Her cookbook Vegetarian Cooking for Everyone *is winning one award after another. No matter what page you open to, the recipe sounds so tempting you want to make it.*

makes 2 to 4 servings

Tofu the way it should be: golden, meaty, and chewy. Use it in stir-fries or serve it with sea salt, soy sauce, or Thai Coconut Marinade and Sauce (page 144).

1 pound Chinese-style firm tofu
2 tablespoons peanut oil
Salt

Drain, and blot the tofu with paper towels. Cut it into 3/4-inch cubes. Heat the oil in a medium nonstick skillet over fairly high heat. Add the tofu, and fry until golden. It takes several minutes to color, so let it cook undisturbed while you do something else; then come back and turn the pieces. Although it takes on color, don't let the tofu get dry and hard. Drain briefly on paper towels; then slide onto a heated serving dish and salt lightly or to taste.

Thai Coconut Marinade and Sauce (v)

Deborah Madison

Vegetarian Cooking for Everyone (Broadway Books, 1997)

makes about 3/4 cup

Brush half the sauce over drained tofu. Marinate tofu for at least 60 minutes. Grill or broil, and serve the remaining marinade as a sauce.

- 1 tablespoon finely chopped ginger
- 5 garlic cloves
- 1/2 cup chopped cilantro
- 1/2 cup unsweetened coconut milk
- 1 1/2 tablespoons soy sauce or 1 tablespoon mushroom sauce
- 2 tablespoons roasted peanut oil
- 2 tablespoons brown sugar
- 1 to 2 teaspoons Thai green curry paste or 2 serrano chiles, chopped
- 2 shallots or 1 medium bunch scallions, including 1 inch of the greens, finely diced

Puree or pound all the ingredients, except the shallots, into a paste. Add the shallots.

Caramelized Golden Tofu (v)

Deborah Madison
Vegetarian Cooking for Everyone (Broadway Books, 1997)

makes about 1½ cups

Deborah credits chef Barbara Tropp for inspiring this recipe. It transforms the Golden Tofu (page 143) into richly lacquered pieces that are delicious in stir-fries and with Chinese noodles. Cut it into triangles, about ½ inch thick, and serve with slivered scallions and toasted sesame seeds.

2 tablespoons soy sauce
3½ tablespoons light brown sugar
Peanut oil for cooking
1 recipe Golden Tofu (page 143)

1. Mix the soy sauce and sugar in a small bowl.
2. Heat a wok or heavy skillet over high heat, add 1 tablespoon of the peanut oil used to fry the tofu or use fresh oil, and swirl it around the wok. When hot, add the soy mixture; reduce the heat to medium, and add the Golden Tofu. Toss well; simmer 2 minutes. Add 3 tablespoons water, and cook until the sauce coats the tofu with a syrupy glaze. Turn off the heat. Let cool in the syrup 10 minutes; then transfer to a serving dish.

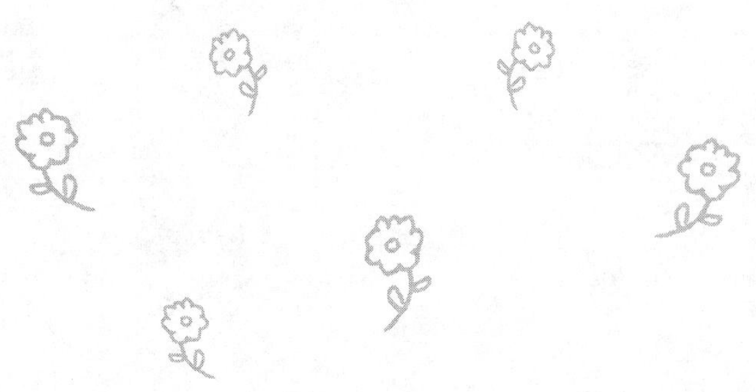

Chile con Queso

Recipe courtesy of *Saveur* magazine

makes 6 servings

You know that rubbery processed cheese you get when you order a plate of nachos? Like melted Tex-Mex Silly Putty? Here's an authentic recipe from the L & J Cafe in El Paso that's real cheese, real spices, real good.

6 fresh Anaheim chiles
2 tablespoons vegetable oil
1 yellow onion, chopped
2 garlic cloves, chopped
1 pound white Cheddar cheese, grated
1 tablespoon sour cream
Tortilla chips

1. Char the chiles over a flame or under the broiler, turning to blacken all over. Place in a paper bag, close, and steam 15 minutes. Rub off the skin and remove the stems. Slice open, scrape out the veins and seeds, and coarsely chop.
2. Heat the oil in a saucepan over medium heat, add the onion and garlic; cook until translucent, about 20 minutes. Add the chiles, and cook another 10 minutes. Reduce the heat to medium-low, and add the cheese; cook, stirring constantly, until melted, about 5 minutes. Stir in the sour cream. Serve immediately with the tortilla chips.

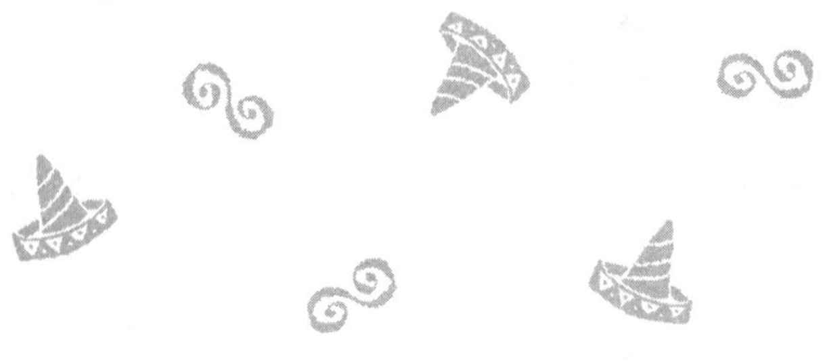

Enchiladas Nortenas (Stacked Cheese Enchiladas)

Recipe courtesy of *Saveur* magazine

makes 4 servings

Forget sixteen candles—celebrate a special occasion with sixteen fire-crackers; hot cheese and chile tortillas, all stacked up like a fantastic south-of-the-border birthday cake.

for the red chile sauce

20 dried New Mexico red chiles
2 garlic cloves, crushed
1 small yellow onion, chopped
1 teaspoon ground cumin
Salt
1 teaspoon sugar (optional)

for the enchiladas

1 1/2 pounds white Cheddar cheese, grated
1 small yellow onion, diced
Corn oil
16 white corn tortillas
1/2 cup crumbled queso fresco (or mild feta)

1. To make the sauce, wash the chiles and remove the stems, seeds, and veins. Bring a pot of water to boil. Add the chiles, cover, and remove from the heat. Soak until soft, about 1 hour; drain, reserving the soaking water.
2. Place the chiles, garlic, chopped onion, and 2 cups of soaking water in a blender or food processor. Puree until smooth. Thin with more soaking water if the sauce is too thick.
3. Strain the sauce into a large saucepan suitable for dipping tortillas. Add the cumin, season to taste with the salt; simmer, uncovered,

over low heat for 10 minutes. If the sauce tastes bitter, add the sugar. Cover to keep warm.

4. To make the enchiladas, combine the Cheddar cheese and diced onion in a small mixing bowl. Heat 1 inch of oil in a large skillet. Fry the tortillas one at a time until the edges are crisp, about 30 seconds. Drain on paper towels.
5. To assemble, ladle some sauce in the center of a plate. Dip a tortilla into the sauce and place it on the plate; cover with ½ cup of the cheese mixture; repeat twice, and top with a fourth dipped tortilla. Keep warm in low oven, and assemble the other plates. When ready to serve, spoon a bit more sauce over each enchilada and top with queso fresco.

Tofu and Tender Vegetable Stir-Fry with Garlic-Basil Sauce (v)

Melissa Hamilton

makes 4 servings

Once you've assembled everything, cooking a stir-fry goes really fast. This one, with its exotic mix of pungent and tangy and green is particularly rich and satisfying.

for the garlic-basil sauce

- 3 medium garlic cloves, minced
- 2 tablespoons minced ginger
- ¼ cup chopped fresh basil leaves
- ¼ cup soy sauce
- 3 tablespoons vegetable stock
- 2 teaspoons balsamic vinegar
- 1 teaspoon Asian sesame oil
- ½ small fresh red chile, stemmed and chopped fine

for the stir-fry

- 3 tablespoons canola oil
- 1 pound firm or extra-firm tofu, drained and cut into 1-inch cubes
- 1/2 pound shiitake mushrooms, stemmed and sliced
- 6 medium scallions, white part cut into 1-inch lengths, green part cut into 1/4-inch lengths
- 1 medium onion, peeled and cut into 8 pieces
- 2 red bell peppers, cut lengthwise into 1/4-inch strips
- 2 teaspoons cornstarch dissolved in 1/4 cup cold water
- 1 recipe Basic Brown Rice (page 110) or 3 cups cooked white rice (optional)

1. To make sauce, combine all the sauce ingredients in a small bowl. Set aside.
2. To make the stir-fry, set a large skillet or wok over high heat, and add 1 tablespoon of the canola oil. When the oil is shimmering hot, throw in the tofu and cook, stirring several times, until browned lightly on all sides. Transfer the tofu to a medium bowl; cover to keep warm. Add the remaining 2 tablespoons of the canola oil to the skillet; when shimmering hot, add the mushrooms, white part of the scallions, and onion; stir-fry 2 minutes. Toss in the bell pepper; stir-fry until just tender; then add to the tofu.
3. Return the skillet to the heat. Pour in the sauce and the cornstarch mixture. Cook until somewhat thickened and the garlic and ginger are no longer raw, 30 to 60 seconds. Quickly return the tofu and vegetables to the skillet, add the green part of the scallions, and toss to heat through. Serve immediately with rice, if desired.

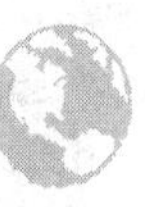

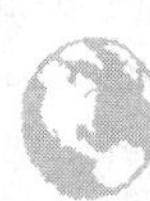

Grilled Fresh Mozzarella Sandwiches with Olive Paste and Roasted Red Peppers

Melissa Hamilton

makes 2 sandwiches

Grown-up grilled cheese, bursting with sophisticated flavors. When it comes to mozzarella, the fresher the better. The fresh mozzarella in water is by far superior to the refrigerator-case variety. Local Italian markets are always a good source. Use smoked mozzarella, if you want.

4 teaspoons prepared olive paste
4 slices European-style country bread
3 ounces fresh mozzarella, grated on the large holes of a box grater (about 1 cup, lightly packed)
2 ounces prepared roasted red peppers cut into 1/2-inch strips
Freshly milled black pepper
2 tablespoons extra-virgin olive oil
1 small garlic clove

1. Heat a heavy 12-inch skillet over low to medium-low heat.
2. Spread 1 teaspoon prepared olive paste on each slice of bread. Sprinkle two bread slices evenly with half the cheese; top each with half the roasted pepper strips and a few grinds of black pepper; cover with the remaining cheese and slices of bread.
3. Brush the sandwich tops completely with half the olive oil; place the sandwiches, oiled side down, in the skillet. Brush the remaining side of each sandwich completely with the remaining oil. Cook until crisp and deep golden brown, 5 to 10 minutes per side, flipping the sandwiches back to the first side to reheat and crisp, about 15 seconds. Rub the toasted sandwiches with the raw clove of garlic. Serve immediately.

Pasta

★ ★ ★ ★ ★

Bucatini with Oven-Baked Tomatoes

Giuliano Hazan

The Classic Pasta Cookbook (Dorling Kindersley, 1997)

If Matthew Kenney is an empire, Giuliano Hazan is a dynasty. His mother, Marcella, and his father, Victor, are the standard-bearers of all that is glorious about Italian food and wine. Giuliano has inherited this gift, and his cookbook is full of simple pasta recipes that produce complex and irresistible flavors.

makes enough to sauce 1 pound of pasta

Tomatoes that bake for an hour transform themselves into a sauce that then takes just a minute to prepare. Giuliano says that the sauce is good with almost any pasta.

1 pound bucatini
3/4 pound fresh, ripe plum tomatoes
1 tablespoon finely chopped garlic
2 tablespoons finely chopped flat-leaf parsley
Salt and freshly milled black pepper
1/3 cup extra-virgin olive oil
1 tablespoon salt
2 tablespoons freshly grated Pecorino Romano cheese
1/4 cup freshly grated Parmigiano-Reggiano cheese

1. Preheat the oven to 350°F.
2. Cut the tomatoes in half lengthwise, remove the seeds, and place in a baking pan with the cut side up. Sprinkle the garlic and parsley into the cavities, and season with salt and pepper to taste. Drizzle the olive oil over the tomatoes. Bake about 1 hour, until the tomatoes have shriveled slightly and begun to brown at the edges. Save the oil from the pan. You can prepare the tomatoes ahead of time; cover and refrigerate.
3. Bring 4 quarts of water to a boil in a large saucepan or pot, add the salt, and drop in the pasta all at once, stirring until the strands are submerged. Cook until al dente, about 8 minutes.
4. When the tomatoes are cool enough to handle, scrape the flesh away from the skin with a knife. Discard the skins, and coarsely chop the flesh. Put the chopped tomatoes and the reserved oil into a saucepan over a medium-low heat. Stir from time to time while the pasta cooks.
5. Drain the pasta, and toss with the sauce and the cheeses. Serve at once.

Spaghetti with Fresh Tomatoes, Herbs, and Mozzarella

Giuliano Hazan

The Classic Pasta Cookbook (Dorling Kindersley, 1997)

makes enough to sauce 1 pound of pasta, about 3–4 cups

This is strictly a summer recipe—an "uncooked" sauce that works with garden-fresh plum tomatoes and herbs. The ingredients are simply scalded in hot oil before being tossed with the pasta.

1 pound spaghetti
1 teaspoon salt
2 pounds fresh, ripe plum tomatoes, peeled, seeded, and cut into 1/4-inch dice
8 ounces whole-milk Italian mozzarella, cut into 1/4-inch dice
2 tablespoons chopped fresh basil leaves
2 tablespoons chopped fresh oregano leaves
2 tablespoons chopped fresh marjoram leaves
1 tablespoon chopped fresh thyme leaves
Salt and freshly milled black pepper
1/2 cup extra-virgin olive oil

1. Bring 4 quarts of water to a boil in a large saucepan or pot, add the salt, and drop in the pasta all at once, stirring until the strands are submerged. Cook until molto al dente (about 30 seconds before al dente), 8 minutes.
2. Put the tomatoes, mozzarella, and all the herbs in a serving bowl large enough to accommodate the cooked pasta. Season with salt and pepper to taste and mix well.
3. Heat the olive oil until it is smoking hot and pour it over the tomato mixture.
4. Drain the pasta, and add to the tomato mixture. Toss vigorously until the pasta is well coated. Cover the bowl with a plate, let stand 2 minutes to melt the cheese. Serve warm.

Penne with Cauliflower, Tomatoes, and Cream

Giuliano Hazan
The Classic Pasta Cookbook (Dorling Kindersley, 1997)

makes enough to sauce 1 pound of pasta, about 3–4 cups

Pasta doesn't have to be the same old same old. This inspired recipe combines cauliflower and cream in a rich sauce.

- 1 pound penne
- 3/4 pound cauliflower, leaves and stem removed
- 1 teaspoon salt
- 4 tablespoons unsalted butter
- 1/3 cup finely chopped yellow onion
- 1/4 teaspoon red pepper flakes
- 1 pound fresh, ripe plum tomatoes, peeled, seeded, and cut into 1/2-inch dice
- 3/4 cup heavy cream
- 1/2 cup freshly grated Parmigiano-Reggiano cheese

1. Cook the cauliflower in abundant unsalted boiling water until tender. When cool enough to handle, cut it into 3/4-inch pieces.
2. Bring 4 quarts of water to boil in large saucepan or pot, add 1 teaspoon salt, and drop the pasta in all at once, stirring well. Cook until al dente, about 8 minutes.
3. Melt the butter in a large skillet over medium heat. Add the onion; cook until softened and golden.
4. Add the red pepper flakes and the cauliflower, and sprinkle with salt, to taste. Sauté until the cauliflower is lightly browned, 8 to 10 minutes. Stir in the tomatoes; cook for 1 minute.
5. Pour the cream into the skillet; cook until reduced by half.
6. Drain the pasta, and toss it with the sauce, adding the cheese. Taste for salt and serve at once.

Cart Wheels with Bell Peppers and Onions (v)

Giuliano Hazan

The Classic Pasta Cookbook (Dorling Kindersley, 1997)

makes enough to sauce 1 pound of pasta, about 3–4 cups

Why eat spaghetti when you can have happy little pasta cart wheels? Why have a plain sauce when you can have one that's red and green and sunny yellow? Giuliano says to peel the peppers. Don't tell him, but when we're in a hurry, we don't. Try this sauce with almost any small pasta shape.

- 1 pound cart wheels
- 1/3 cup extra-virgin olive oil
- 2 cups thinly sliced yellow onions
- 2 red bell peppers, peeled and cut lengthwise into 1/4-inch-wide strips
- 2 yellow bell peppers, peeled and cut lengthwise into 1/4-inch-wide strips
- 1 cup canned whole peeled tomatoes, with the juice, coarsely chopped
- Salt and freshly milled black pepper
- Pinch red pepper flakes
- 1 tablespoon finely chopped flat-leaf parsley
- 1 teaspoon salt

1. Put the olive oil and onions in a large skillet over low heat. Cook, stirring occasionally, until wilted and golden.
2. Turn the heat up to medium, and add the red and yellow bell peppers; cook, stirring frequently, until softened slightly, 2 to 3 minutes.
3. Stir in the tomatoes and juice, season with salt and black pepper to taste, and add the red pepper. Stir well; cook until the tomatoes have reduced and separated from the oil, about 20 minutes.
4. Add the parsley, stir for about 30 seconds, and remove from the

heat. Set aside. You can prepare the sauce ahead of time up to this point and refrigerate it.

5. Bring 4 quarts of water to a boil in a large saucepan or pot, add 1 teaspoon of salt, and drop in the pasta all at once, stirring well. Cook until al dente, about 8 minutes.
6. When the pasta is almost done, return the sauce to medium heat.
7. Drain the pasta, and toss with the sauce. Taste for salt and serve at once.

"Mange Tout" Sesame Noodles (v)

Rozanne Gold
Little Meals (Villard, 1993)

makes 4 servings for a light main course

You know how sometimes you'd rather order two appetizers than one main course? Rozanne's books feature smaller dishes you can happily build a meal on. This one is everyone's favorite Chinese take-out: sesame noodles topped with chilled snow peas.

for the noodles

- 3/4 pound linguine
- 1 1/2 tablespoons soy sauce
- 2 tablespoons toasted sesame oil
- 1 tablespoon rice wine vinegar
- 1 tablespoon honey
- 1/2 tablespoon toasted white sesame seeds
- 1-inch piece of ginger, chopped
- 1 scallion, chopped
- 1 garlic clove, halved
- 1/4 cup peanut butter
- 1/4 teaspoon hot sauce

for the garnish

- 1/2 pound snow peas, blanched, chilled, and julienned
- 1/4 cup chopped scallions
- 2 teaspoons black sesame seeds

1. Cook the linguine in a large pot of boiling water until done. Drain, and rinse under cool water. Drain again. Reserve.
2. Place the remaining noodle ingredients in a food processor fitted with the steel blade. Process until very smooth. Add 2 tablespoons of water to dilute; the color will lighten.
3. Mix the noodles with sauce. Divide evenly onto four plates, and garnish with snow peas, 1/4 cup of scallions, and black sesame seeds. Serve with chopsticks just for fun.

Farfalle with Broccoli, Broccoli Butter Sauce

Rozanne Gold
Little Meals (Villard, 1998)

makes 4 servings for a light main course

With only three ingredients and four baby steps, this broccoli and pasta dish is a winner.

- 8 ounces farfalle (bow tie) pasta
- 1 large head broccoli (1 pound)
- Salt and freshly milled black pepper
- 3 tablespoons butter, cold and cut into small pieces

1. Cut the broccoli into florets, leaving only 1/2 inch of the stem. Reserve.

2. Peel the remaining stems and cut them into 1-inch pieces. Cook, covered, in 1¼ cups of salted water until very soft, about 25 minutes. Transfer the stems and water to a blender; puree until very smooth. Add the butter and blend. Add a little extra water, if necessary, to make a smooth sauce. Add salt and pepper to taste, and transfer to a small pot.
3. Cook the pasta in salted boiling water for 10 minutes. Add the broccoli florets, and cook until tender, 3 to 4 minutes. Drain.
4. Heat the sauce gently and serve over the pasta and broccoli.

★ ★ ★ ★ ★

Over-Stuffed Baked Potato

(V, if made without the dairy products)

Stephanie Pierson
(South Salem, New York)

makes 1 serving

When all else fails, there's almost always a potato in the pantry and some vegetables in your refrigerator. And with these humble ingredients you can make a snack, dinner, or lunch that everyone loves. Sometimes we make this stuffed potato the night before, refrigerate it, and reheat it the next night. It's not quite as good that way, but it still beats a frozen burrito or our fourth consecutive night of take-out vegetable pizza.

1 baking potato
Handful of raw vegetables
About 1 tablespoon butter or olive oil
About 1/4 cup cream or soy milk
Salt and freshly milled black pepper
Cheddar cheese or soy cheese

1. Preheat the oven to 400°F. Prick the potato, so it doesn't explode, and bake 1 hour, until tender.
2. Meanwhile, cut up some vegetables into little pieces and steam them. A handful of broccoli florets and diced carrots or green beans are good.
3. When the potato is done, let it cool; then cut in half lengthwise, and scoop out the potato, leaving the shell intact.

4. In a saucepan, mash the potato with a little butter and cream. Stir in the cooked vegetables; add salt and pepper to taste.
5. Spoon the potato mixture back into the shell. Sprinkle the top with some cheese. Reheat the potato in the oven for a few minutes.

Tommy's Rice and Beans (v)

Chris Schlesinger and John Willoughby
License to Grill (William Morrow, 1997)

The dynamic duo of Chris Schlesinger and John Willoughby is the Fred Astaire and Ginger Rogers of the food circuit. Aside from their separate gigs (Chris co-owns and runs two Boston restaurants, John edits a food magazine), together they write terrific cookbooks, run cooking classes, and host a show on the TV Food Network. A funny, smart, talented team.

makes 4 servings

Tommy who? Chris and John explain: "This classic Latin American dish is that rare bird, a completely healthful vegetarian meal that appeals to the taste buds of teenagers. Or at least it appeals to the buds of Tommy, a teenager who lives in the apartment above one of us and is the nephew of the other one. Tommy prefers his rice and beans cooked separately, rather than together, and likes lots of garlic and only a few bell peppers in the mix; so that's how we make it here. For some reason, it has almost as high an appeal rating as pizza and chips, those quintessential meatless teenage favorites."

- 1 tablespoon olive oil
- 1 onion, diced small
- 1 tablespoon minced garlic
- 1 roasted red bell pepper, thinly sliced
- One 16-ounce can black beans or 2 cups cooked black beans
- 1/4 cup white vinegar

5 to 10 dashes Tabasco sauce or other hot red pepper sauce
$1/4$ cup roughly chopped cilantro
3 cups cooked long-grain rice
Salt and freshly milled black pepper

1. In a large sauté pan, heat the oil over medium-high heat until hot but not smoking. Add the onion, and sauté, stirring occasionally, until transparent, 5 to 7 minutes. Add the garlic and roasted pepper, and sauté, stirring occasionally, for an additional 2 minutes.
2. Add the black beans, vinegar, and Tabasco sauce. Bring the mixture to a boil; reduce the heat to low, cover, and simmer 5 minutes.
3. Add the cilantro and rice; mix well. Season to taste with the salt and black pepper. Serve accompanied by additional hot pepper sauce.

Cherry Tomato Boboli

Rozanne Gold
Little Meals (Villard, 1993)

makes 4 servings for a light main course

Besides making your own and take-out, here's another pizza option. Boboli crusts from the supermarket with a fresh tomato topping.

3 tablespoons vegetable oil
$1/4$ cup finely chopped onion
$1\,1/2$ pounds cherry tomatoes
$1\,1/4$ tablespoons dried tarragon
2 tablespoons cider vinegar
1 tablespoon apple jelly
Salt and pepper to taste
Two 7-inch Bobolis
$1/2$ cup shredded Asiago cheese

1. Preheat the oven to 500°F.
2. Heat the oil in a large nonstick skillet; add the onion and sauté until soft but not brown.
3. Add the tomatoes; cook over medium heat until they get soft and burst open, 10 to 15 minutes.
4. Add the tarragon, vinegar, and jelly; season with salt and pepper to taste. Cook over high heat, pressing down on tomatoes, until the liquid has thickened, 5 minutes.
5. Spread the mixture over tops of the Boboli crusts, and sprinkle evenly with the cheese. Bake on an ungreased cookie sheet for 8 minutes. Cut in half and serve.

Roasted Mushrooms with Brown Rice Gravy (v)

Angelica Kitchen
(New York City)

makes 6 servings

Now you don't need to make a meat loaf to have glossy, rich, homemade gravy. This veggie version is also wonderful spooned on top of mashed potatoes or a bowl of kasha.

for the gravy

- 1/3 cup plus 1 tablespoon brown rice flour
- 3 1/2 tablespoons canola oil
- 5 tablespoons naturally brewed shoyu or tamari
- 2 tablespoons minced fresh herbs, such as thyme, sage, rosemary, or tarragon

for the mushrooms

10 ounces mushrooms, such as shiitake, cremini, or chanterelle, stems trimmed
1 tablespoon olive oil
1 tablespoon minced garlic
Pinch sea salt
Pinch freshly milled black pepper

1. To make the gravy, combine the flour and canola oil in a 2 quart, heavy-bottomed saucepan. Stir with a wooden spoon over medium heat until toasty and lightly browned, 5 to 7 minutes.
2. Whisk in 3 cups of water. Add the shoyu and herbs. Bring to a boil; lower the heat and simmer gently for 20 minutes.
3. Preheat the oven to 400°F.
4. Quickly rinse the mushrooms, drain well, and pat dry. Slice into thin pieces and toss with the olive oil, garlic, salt, and pepper.
5. Spread the mushrooms on a greased baking sheet large enough to hold them in a single layer, and roast 20 minutes, stirring occasionally.
6. Stir the mushrooms into the gravy. Serve warm.

Mashed Potatoes with Garlic and Rosemary (v)

Angelica Kitchen
(New York City)

makes 4 to 6 servings

What are you going to put your Brown Rice Gravy (page 162) on? Creamy Angelica Kitchen mashed potatoes! These are highly evolved and highly delicious: Yukon gold potatoes, fresh rosemary, garlic, and sea salt.

2 pounds yellow fleshed potatoes (such as Yukon gold)
1/3 cup peeled garlic cloves, whole
1 teaspoon fresh rosemary leaves, minced
1 teaspoon salt
6 tablespoons extra-virgin olive oil
Freshly milled black pepper

1. Wash the potatoes. Peel half of them and cut them all into 1-inch cubes; put in a large pot. Add the garlic, rosemary, and salt. Add enough water to cover the potatoes by 1 inch. Bring to a boil over high heat. Lower the heat, cover, and simmer until the potatoes crush easily with the back of a spoon against the side of the pot, 30 to 40 minutes. Drain, reserving the cooking liquid.
2. Add the oil to the potatoes and beat with a wire whisk or wooden spoon, adding enough cooking water to create the desired creaminess. Add the pepper and additional salt to taste.

Kid-Soft Polenta
(V, if made without butter)

Ken Haedrich
Feeding the Healthy Vegetarian Family (Bantam, 1998)

makes 8 servings

Ken, a vegetarian chef who has four vegetarian kids came up with the novel notion of adding cream of wheat to polenta to make it less dense and more kid-friendly.

This polenta needs your undivided attention for 15 to 20 minutes, during which time it should be stirred regularly. The polenta can be eaten warm, spooned onto a plate and topped with tomato sauce or it can be poured into a loaf pan, cooled, chilled overnight, and cut into slices. Hot or cold, you'll want to top it with something: cheese, sautéed vegetables, caramelized onions, sautéed mushrooms, gravy, and tomato sauce are some ideas.

- 1 scant teaspoon salt
- 1 cup fine yellow cornmeal
- 1/2 cup regular cream of wheat cereal (not instant)
- 1 tablespoon unsalted butter or olive oil

1. Butter a large loaf pan and set it aside.
2. Put 4½ cups of cold water and the salt in a large saucepan. Whisk in the cornmeal and cream of wheat. Cook over medium heat, whisking often. When the cereal reaches a boil, reduce the heat slightly and continue to cook, stirring often with a wooden spoon, for about 10 minutes. If it becomes almost too thick to stir, add extra water a tablespoon or so at a time.
3. After 10 minutes, when it is quite thick, stir in the butter; then scrape the polenta into the loaf pan. Cool on a rack to room temperature; then cover and refrigerate overnight. When the polenta is thoroughly chilled, run a knife around the edge, and invert onto a cutting board. Slice as needed, brush with oil, and sauté or grill.

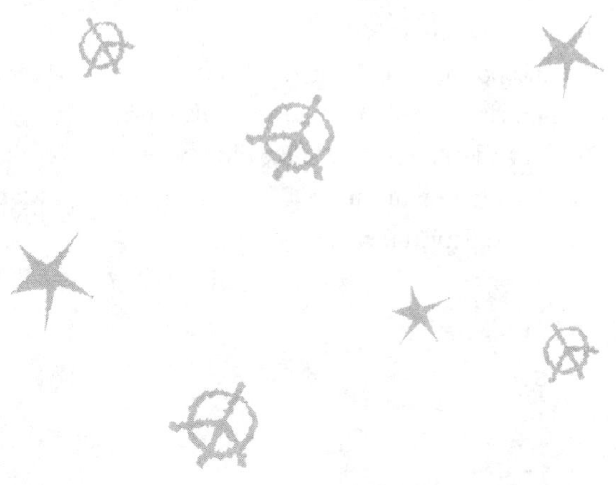

Dry-Curry Sweet Potatoes (v)

Rozanne Gold
Recipes 1-2-3 (Viking, 1996)

makes 4 servings

Sweet potatoes that, for once, aren't achingly sweet. These have a slight Indian accent.

- 1½ pounds medium to large sweet potatoes
- 2 tablespoons good-quality curry powder
- 1 teaspoon salt
- 2 tablespoons olive oil

1. Preheat the oven to 400°F.
2. Peel the potatoes, and cut them into 1-inch chunks. Place in a medium-sized shallow ungreased casserole. Sprinkle the curry powder and salt and drizzle the olive oil evenly over the top.
3. Bake 45 minutes, turning once or twice so they brown evenly and don't stick. Serve immediately.

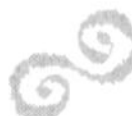 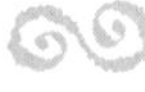 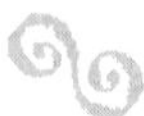

Overnight Tabbouleh with Melted Feta Cheese

Rozanne Gold
Little Meals (Villard, 1993)

makes 4 to 6 servings for a light main course

This cracked wheat salad is an overnight sensation. Before you go to bed, get all the ingredients ready (chop, chop, chop, chop, chop, chop, squeeze), and this dish will make itself.

- 1/2 pound bulgur wheat
- 1/4 cup sesame seeds
- 1/2 cup finely chopped carrot
- 1/2 cup finely chopped celery
- 1/4 cup finely chopped onion
- 1 tomato, chopped
- 1/2 cup finely chopped red pepper
- 1/2 cup finely chopped green pepper
- 1 cup canned tomato juice
- 1/2 cup fresh lemon juice
- 1/3 cup plus 2 tablespoons extra-virgin olive oil
- 2 teaspoons fresh thyme leaves
- 3/4 teaspoon salt
- 1/2 cup all-purpose flour
- 1/2 pound feta or kasseri cheese, cut into eight to twelve 2- × 1- × 1/2-inch rectangles
- Sprigs fresh thyme for garnish (optional)

1. In a large bowl, combine the bulgur, sesame seeds, vegetables, and juices. Add 1/3 cup of the olive oil, 1 cup cold water, the thyme and the salt. Mix well; cover and refrigerate overnight.
2. Remove the tabbouleh from refrigerator, and mix well. Divide evenly onto four to six plates, and mound into circles.

3. Heat 2 tablespoons of the olive oil in a nonstick skillet. Lightly flour the cheese rectangles, and brown 1 to 2 minutes on each side. Put two pieces of cheese on top of each portion of tabbouleh. Garnish with thyme sprigs, if desired.

Asparagus in Ambush

Larry Forgione
An American Place (New York City)

makes 4 servings

Asparagus in Ambush (a name rivaled only by Pigs-in-a-blanket) was originally a popular fifties cocktail hors d'oeuvre. Larry has kept the essence of this traditional finger food and turned it into a sensational nineties wrap.

Four 10-inch flour tortillas
2 tablespoons Sun-Dried Tomato Pesto (recipe below)
4 ounces Brie (or other cheese) cut into 8 long, thin slices
24 asparagus spears, trimmed, blanched al dente, and cooled
Freshly milled black pepper
1 ounce lightly toasted pine nuts or other nuts (chopped)
Olive oil for brushing.

1. Preheat oven to 300°F.
2. In the oven, warm each of the tortillas so they are pliable. Remove from oven and spread each with one tablespoon Sun-Dried Tomato Pesto. Add a slice of Brie and then six asparagus spears, three facing the opposite way. Season with a little black pepper, sprinkle with some pine nuts, and top with the second slice of brie. Fold one side over the asparagus spears and Brie. Fold in the two sides and wrap tightly.
3. Place the asparagus in ambush on a lightly oiled cookie sheet and brush each lightly with oil. Warm in the oven 8 to 10 minutes. Serve with additional pesto, as desired.

Sun-Dried Tomato Pesto (v)

Larry uses this as a spread. But if you thin it with a little warm water, this pesto is also excellent as a simple pasta sauce.

- 4 ounces sun-dried tomatoes packed in olive oil
- 4 tablespoons chopped fresh basil leaves
- 1 tablespoon chopped garlic

Puree all ingredients in a blender or small food processor fitted with the steel blade.

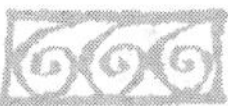

Braised Collard Greens and Black-Eyed Peas (v)

Blanche's Organic Café (New York City)

makes 4 servings

This version of the traditional Southern dish condenses the cooking time without short-changing the flavor. To make it even quicker, use canned peas. If you can't find collard greens, use kale instead.

- 1 tablespoon olive oil
- 1/2 cup thinly sliced onion
- 2 garlic cloves, minced
- 1 bunch collard greens, stems removed, washed and chopped coarse (12 cups)
- 1 cup cooked black-eyed peas
- 1 cup vegetable stock
- Salt and freshly milled black pepper
- Hot pepper sauce (optional)

1. In a large skillet or Dutch oven, heat the olive oil over medium heat; add the onion and sauté until translucent, 3 to 4 minutes.
2. Raise the heat to medium-high, add the garlic and collard greens (you may need to add them in two batches), and cook, stirring and turning the greens frequently, until the greens are wilted, about 6 minutes.
3. Add the black-eyed peas, stock, and salt and pepper to taste. Bring to a boil; reduce the heat to low, and simmer, stirring occasionally, until greens are dark green and tender and the liquid has reduced a bit, about 15 minutes more. Adjust the seasonings, adding a few dashes of hot pepper sauce if desired.

Grilled Sweet Potato with Cilantro Pesto (v)

Blanche's Organic Café (New York City)

makes 4 servings

A vibrant and unexpected side dish—a pairing of familiar and exotic flavors. While these are better grilled (isn't everything?), you can roast them in the oven instead.

- 4 medium sweet potatoes, washed and dried
- 1/2 cup cilantro, washed and thoroughly dried
- 1/2 cup parsley, washed and thoroughly dried
- 1/4 cup toasted pine nuts or walnuts
- 1 garlic clove, chopped
- 1 tablespoon soy Parmesan or dairy Parmesan cheese
- 1/2 cup extra-virgin olive oil, plus more for brushing

1. Preheat the oven to 400°F. Preheat the grill.
2. Prick the potatoes a few times with a fork, place on foil-lined baking pan, and roast 30 to 45 minutes, until almost tender.
3. In a blender or small food processor fitted with the steel blade, combine the cilantro, parsley, pine nuts, garlic, and cheese. With machine running, slowly pour in the olive oil, blending until mixture is pureed.
4. When potatoes are cool enough to handle, peel off the skins, and cut into quarters lengthwise. Brush with the olive oil, and grill until well marked on all sides and the potatoes are cooked through. Serve warm with the cilantro pesto drizzled over top.

Honey-Mustard Fried Tempeh (v)

Blanche's Organic Café (New York City)

makes 4 servings

This is great party food, and the only trick is that you have to serve it as soon as it's done.

- 1/4 cup tamari or shoyu
- 1/4 teaspoon onion powder
- 1/4 teaspoon garlic powder
- One 8-ounce package tempeh, cut into 8 triangular wedges
- 1/2 cup Dijon mustard
- 1/4 cup honey
- 1/2 cup all-purpose flour
- 1/2 cup bread crumbs
- 1/4 cup vegetable oil

1. In a nonreactive, shallow dish large enough to hold the tempeh in a single layer, combine ⅓ cup water and the tamari, onion powder, and garlic powder. Place the tempeh in marinade, cover with plastic wrap and refrigerate for 1 hour and up to 4 hours, turning once or twice.
2. Combine the mustard and honey in a blender on high speed. Transfer half the honey-mustard dipping sauce to a plate and the other half to a small bowl for dipping at the table.
3. Put the flour and bread crumbs on two separate plates. Remove the tempeh from the marinade, dip each piece into the flour, then the honey-mustard sauce, and then the bread crumbs.
4. Heat the oil in a large skillet over medium-high heat. Fry the tempeh until golden, turning to cook on all sides. Remove the pieces from skillet, drain on paper towels, and serve warm with honey-mustard dipping sauce.

Lemon Tofu Cheesecake (v)

Angelica Kitchen (New York City)

makes 10 to 12 servings

Lemony, luscious, rich, refreshing—this is one of those recipes that make a vegetarian feel he or she isn't giving up anything. Tofu substitutes nicely for cream. Want to gild the lily? Glaze the cake with fresh strawberries or blueberries. The agar flakes are available at most health food stores.

for the crust

1 1/2 cups pastry flour
1/2 teaspoon baking powder
1/2 teaspoon cinnamon
6 tablespoons canola oil
6 tablespoons maple syrup
1/2 teaspoon plus pinch salt

for the filling

2 pounds firm tofu
1/3 cup canola oil
1 1/2 cups maple syrup
1/2 teaspoon salt
1/2 teaspoon minced lemon zest
1/4 cup fresh lemon juice, strained
2 tablespoons vanilla
3 tablespoons agar flakes
2 tablespoons arrowroot powder
3/4 cup plain soy milk
Strawberry Topping (recipe below) or Blueberry Topping (recipe below) (optional)

1. Preheat the oven to 350°F. Oil a 9-inch springform pan.
2. To make the crust, mix together the pastry flour, baking powder, and cinnamon in one bowl and the canola oil, maple syrup, and salt in another.
3. Mix the wet ingredients into the dry ingredients until no dry particles remain. Press into bottom of the prepared pan.
4. Bake about 15 minutes, until the crust is golden. Cool completely.
5. To make the filling, press the tofu for at least 30 minutes to remove the excess water. Blend in a food processor with the canola oil, maple syrup, salt, lemon juice, and vanilla. Process until very creamy. Alternately, use a blender, and blend in two batches. Add the lemon zest.
6. In a small saucepan, dissolve the agar in 1 cup of water over medium heat, stirring frequently. Simmer slowly, until the flakes completely disappear. In a small bowl, dissolve arrowroot in the soy milk. Pour over the agar mixture, stirring continuously until it begins to bubble and has thickened considerably. Add to the tofu mixture and process until everything has completely melded.
7. Pour the filling into the prepared crust. Place in the refrigerator to set, about 1 hour. Run a knife around the cheesecake before releasing the sides of the pan. Top with Strawberry or Blueberry Topping, if desired.

Strawberry Topping (V)

makes 2 cups

- 2 pints strawberries, hulled and sliced thin
- 2 tablespoons maple syrup
- 1 tablespoon fresh lemon juice
- 1/2 teaspoon vanilla

Combine all the ingredients. Spoon over the chilled cheesecake and serve.

Blueberry Topping (v)

makes 2 cups

1 pint blueberries
1/2 cup apple cider
2 tablespoons maple syrup
1 teaspoon vanilla
2 tablespoons arrowroot dissolved in 1/2 cup apple juice

Bring the blueberries, cider, maple syrup, and vanilla to a boil in a small pot. When mixture reaches a boil, add the arrowroot mixture, and stir until thickened and the liquid has cleared. Cool completely before spooning over the chilled cheesecake.

Chocolate Devastation Cake (v)

Mark Feldman
Mrs. Green's Natural Market
(Eastchester and Mt. Kisco, New York)

Mark Feldman, who does a tremendous amount of vegetarian cooking and baking and catering, supplies Mrs. Green's Natural Market with most of their prepared food. Thanks to Mark, the refrigerator case is filled with jewel-colored salads and savory stews and wraps. Thanks to Phoebe and our constant expeditions to Mrs. Green's, our refrigerator looks like homage to Mark.

makes 6 to 8 servings

Happy birthday, dear vegan! Here's the ultimate truly stupendous nondairy chocolate birthday cake. Mark ended the copy of the recipe he gave us with "Enjoy!" You will.

dry ingredients

- 2 cups all-purpose flour
- 1/2 cup cocoa powder
- 1 tablespoon aluminum-free baking powder
- 1 teaspoon baking soda

wet ingredients

- 1/2 pound extra-firm tofu, drained and cubed
- 1 1/4 cups maple syrup, grade B
- 1 1/4 cups canola oil
- 3/4 cup vanilla-flavored soy milk
- 1/4 cup black cherry concentrate
- 1 tablespoon vanilla

Chocolate Icing (below)

1. Preheat the oven to 325°F. Oil and flour two 8-inch springform pans.
2. In a medium bowl, sift together the dry ingredients.
3. In a blender, blend together the wet ingredients, until smooth.
4. Whisk the tofu mixture into the dry ingredients. Pour the batter into the prepared pans. Bake in center of the oven for about 30 minutes, or until a toothpick inserted in the center comes out clean. Remove from the oven and let rest 5 minutes before removing from the sides of the pans. Allow the cakes to cool completely before removing the bottom of the pans. Frost with Chocolate Icing.

Chocolate Icing (V)

- 1 cup cocoa powder
- 1 cup maple syrup
- 1 1/4 sticks soy margarine, softened
- 1 teaspoon vanilla

Toasted sliced almonds, for garnish

Process all the ingredients, except the almonds, in a food processor fitted with the steel blade until silky smooth. Spread about one-third of the icing on top of one of the layers, place the second layer on top, and cover the top and sides of the cake with the remaining icing. Press the almonds onto sides of the cake.

Chocolate Peanut Butter Krispy Rice Treats (v)

Louis Centeri
Blanche's Organic Café (New York City)

makes 20 servings

Chef Louis Centeri figured out how to make a vegan version of the Rice Krispies dessert we all grew up on. And he made it just as gooey and crunchy and yummy. For variety, he likes to substitute different nut butters for the peanut butter and carob chips for the chocolate chips.

2 cups brown rice syrup
1 cup maple syrup
1 cup dairy-free chocolate chips
1 cup peanut butter
1 tablespoon pure vanilla
One 10-ounce box Erewhon Krispy Brown Rice cereal (8 cups)

1. Preheat the oven to 350°F. Oil a 9- × 13-inch baking dish.
2. In a medium-sized, nonreactive, heavy-bottomed saucepan, bring the brown rice and maple syrups to a slow boil over low heat.
3. Add the chocolate chips, and whisk until melted. Whisk in the peanut butter. When mixture is smooth, remove from the heat, and stir in the vanilla.
4. Place the cereal in a large mixing bowl, and stir in the chocolate–peanut butter mixture. When well combined, spread evenly in the prepared dish; bake 10 minutes. Cool completely before cutting into squares with a sharp knife.

Creamy Peanut Butter and Banana Pudding (v)

Ken Haedrich
Feeding the Healthy Vegetarian Family (Bantam, 1998)

makes 4 servings

Peanut butter and banana take a whirl in the blender together. And a good time is had by all. On a more serious culinary note, Ken Haedrich explains: "When you puree tofu with the right ingredients, you get a smooth, creamy dessert very much like a regular dairy-based pudding. But unlike those puddings, this one is not cooked. You just buzz everything right in the blender, pour it into custard cups, chill, and serve. It's that easy. It tastes wonderful plain or dusted with finely chopped peanuts and flaked coconut." If you don't like bananas, you can make a plain peanut butter pudding instead.

- 1/3 cup maple syrup
- 4 tablespoons plain soy milk
- 1/2 ripe medium banana
- 1 teaspoon fresh lemon juice
- 1/2 teaspoon vanilla
- 1/3 cup smooth, natural salted peanut butter
- 1/2 pound firm or extra-firm tofu

1. Put the maple syrup, 2 tablespoons of soy milk, the banana, lemon juice, vanilla, and peanut butter in a blender in the order listed. Cut the tofu into three pieces; working with one piece at a time, squeeze out most of the liquid from each piece using your cupped hands. Crumble all of the tofu. Turn on a blender and gradually add tofu. Gradually add as much of the remaining soy milk as needed to make the pudding smooth; scrape down the sides.
2. Scrape the pudding into ramekins or custard cups. Cover and refrigerate for at least 2 hours before serving.

Fruit Crisp

Brendan Walsh
The Elms Restaurant and Tavern
(Ridgefield, CT)

makes 8 servings

Crisps go into the oven with the fruit on the bottom and a crunchy golden crust on top. They come out of the oven all warm and bubbly and juicy and aromatic. It's a little baking magic that can make even a fruit hater's mouth water. You can make crisps with most of the fruits you have on hand and create your own combos once you get the hang of it.

- 10 cups prepared fruit, see Variations (below) or your own combination
- 2 tablespoons chopped candied ginger or candied orange (optional)
- 1 cup all-purpose flour
- 1 cup packed light brown sugar
- 1/2 cup rolled oats
- 1/4 cup chopped walnuts or other nuts
- 1/2 teaspoon cinnamon
- Pinch salt
- 2 tablespoons unsalted butter, at room temperature, cut into small pieces
- 1/4 cup heavy cream

1. Preheat the oven to 350°F.
2. In a large bowl, toss together the prepared fruit with the candied fruit, if using. Transfer to a 9- × 13- × 2-inch ungreased baking dish; set aside.
3. In a medium bowl, combine the flour, brown sugar, oats, nuts, cinnamon, and salt. With a pastry cutter, fork, or your fingertips, work the butter into the flour mixture. Add the cream and continue mixing until it just comes together in moist lumps.
4. Spread the streusel topping evenly over the fruit. Bake 50 to 60

minutes, until the topping is golden and the fruit juices are thick, syrupy, and bubbling hot. Best served warm.

VARIATIONS: Try 5 cups of 1-inch pieces of banana mixed with 5 cups of halved strawberries. Or 8 cups of 1-inch pieces of peeled pears mixed with 2 cups of raspberries. Another great mix is 8 cups of 1-inch pieces of peeled apple with 2 cups blueberries.

Questions and Answers

With teenagers who are becoming vegetarian, I think the best stance is saying, "Go for it." Just make sure you have the knowledge to back it up.

—David Page, New York restaurant owner and healthy food advocate

question: I've heard that sugar contains animal bones. Is that true?

answer: In some brands of refined sugar, slaughterhouse bones are turned into what amounts to a charcoal filter to help give the sugar its white color. It's hard to know which brands contain bone char, but neither Jack Frost nor Florida Crystal contain any. And you won't find bone char in Turbinado (raw sugar). Bone china, by the way, also contains a small amount of ground-up bone.

★

question: What, exactly, does it mean when it says that a food is "organic"? Also, what's the difference between natural and organic?

answer: We all tend to think that organic refers to food that has been raised or produced with no pesticides or chemicals or additives—essentially, food that's produced more naturally. Actually, the word organic doesn't describe a food at all, it describes a system of growing food. And until recently, except for a few states, there has been no regulation of what that system really means.

Natural is a term that's generally used to describe food that doesn't contain artificial color or flavor. The term *natural* can be used lots of different ways to just suggest healthier, more wholesome food, since there are no regulations to using the term.

Finally, the new National Organic Program will actually set rules and standards for farmers and food processors. The new federal guidelines ensure that farmers don't use synthetic fertilizers or pesticides and that they do use low-environmental-impact farming. "Organic" means it can't have been genetically engineered or irradiated. After virtually ignoring the whole organic food industry for years, the government is not only recognizing it but acknowledging how important it is.

Are organic foods the best way to go? Mostly, a resounding yes, but organic foods aren't guaranteed to be more nutritional than nonorganic foods. *The Yale Guide to Children's Nutrition* points out that some studies of the herbicides used in wheat production have shown that the vitamin content actually increases when the herbicides are used. And organic fertilizers may be a source of bacteria, since they aren't sterilized.

Another drawback can be the price. Food raised organically can cost more than food raised nonorganically because production costs more. The hope is that the easier it is for farmers to grow organic food and the more support they get from the government, the more likely it will be that the quality of the food can be higher and the prices lower. With the incredible success of the organic food industry (sales reached $3.5 billion in 1996) and strong consumer activism, there's every reason to be optimistic.

"I'm very low-key about teenage vegetarianism. When teens come in for routine check-ups, I talk to them about their diets and check their blood. From my experience, I've found that teen vegetarians who eat eggs do better—they're a little healthier."

—Dr. Richard Saphir, clinical professor of pediatrics at Mt. Sinai School of Medicine

★

question: Do vegetarians have to follow the regular Food Pyramid, or is there a special food pyramid for vegetarians?

answer: No, you don't and yes, there is. In 1991, the government replaced the idea of the four basic food groups with the Food Pyramid, which has at the bottom the foods you should eat most of (bread and grains), and at the top the foods you should eat very little of (fats and sweets).

This USDA Food Pyramid makes sense in general; but it doesn't work for vegetarians, and it is useless for vegans because part of the pyramid includes a dairy grouping. Plus vegetarian foods like tofu and meat analogs aren't included as options to meat. Beans and nuts are barely acknowledged in the pyramid, nor is there any way you'd know how much more nutritional they are than the meat and poultry they are grouped with. (Can you say "meat lobby"?)

Soon after the USDA pyramid came out, the Health Connection devised a vegetarian food pyramid, which is an excellent alternative. It shows that dairy can be low-fat or nonfat and indicates that there are nondairy alternatives. It also says "whole grain" bread, not just "bread."

★

question: What do I need to know about pesticides and additives?

answer: The plus side of pesticides is that because of them, more fresh produce is available more cheaply throughout the year. The plus side of additives is how much they can improve the quality, taste, nutrition, and safety of the foods we eat. The bad news is that we are becoming more aware of how harmful many of these chemicals can be.

In general, the risks and benefits of food additives are something you need to address on an individual basis. One additive you're likely to hear about often is *monosodium glutamate* (MSG), a flavor enhancer that is used in lots of Chinese restaurants. Many people ask that their food be made without MSG because they're sensitive to it and experience dizziness, headaches, and nausea when they eat food prepared with it. *Artificial sugars* are another common additive. Some people are leery of sugar substitutes like *saccharin* and *aspartame* (Equal and NutraSweet), but they've been tested over and over by the Food and Drug Administration (FDA) and found to be safe. *Sulfites* are also well-known preservatives you'll find in everything from potato chips to dried fruits. Because of adverse reactions from people who are sulfite-sensitive, sulfites have been closely monitored by the FDA. They're no longer used in restaurant salad bars to keep produce from spoiling, and supermarkets need to label any packaged good that's high in sulfites.

Most important, you should know that the benefits of eating a diet that is high in fruits and vegetables outweighs the risk of the small amounts of pesticides that might be on the food. The consensus is to keep eating that produce but buy organic when you can, especially for fruits and vegetables that are most likely to have pesticide residues.

Vegetarian Food Pyramid

★ ★ ★ ★ ★

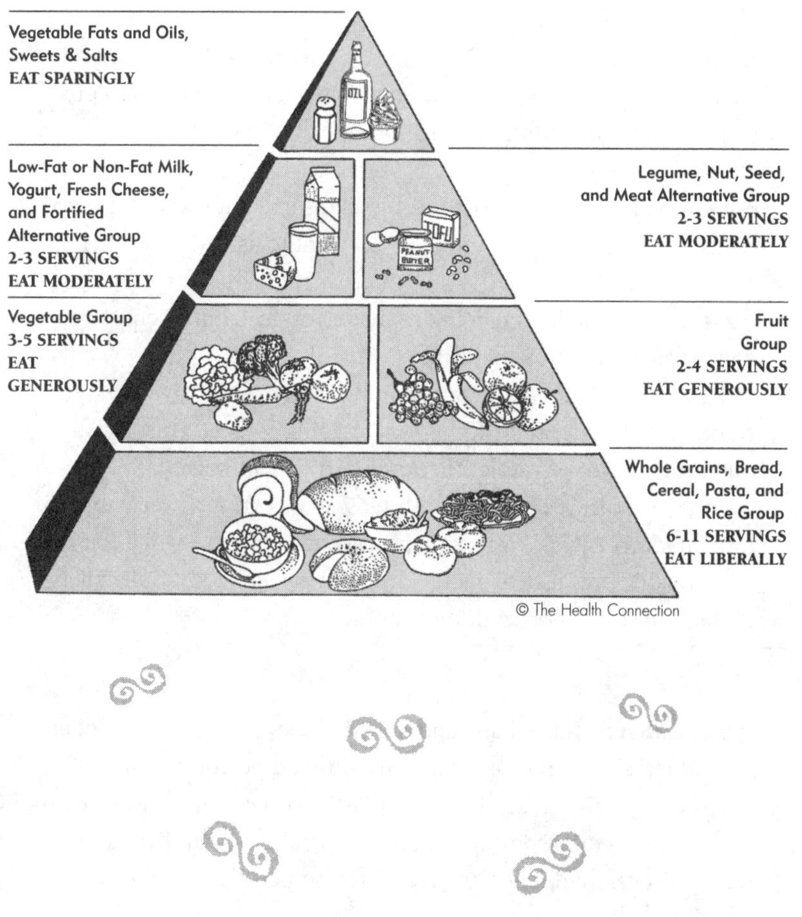

© The Health Connection

Some other tips: the most contaminated fruit you can eat are strawberries. Some of the least contaminated fruits and vegetables—cauliflower, corn, blueberries, carrots, broccoli, and bananas—are also considered best-for-you foods.

Imported produce, especially in places where farming conditions are fairly primitive and not well regulated, is much more likely to be contaminated than is domestic produce.

★

question: Short of not eating strawberries and raspberries at all, especially imported ones, what are you supposed to do to protect yourself from contaminated food?

answer: The government just issued some guidelines for food safety, and they've got a hotline if you want to ask a question. The number is (800) 332–4010. Their new guidelines for preparing fruits and vegetables are going to make you feel a little obsessive-compulsive but here's the drill:

Always wash them under running water. Scrub with a vegetable brush. Even rinse foods you're going to peel. (Just by slicing a melon, for example, the knife can spread bacteria.) Throw out the outer leaves of lettuce. If the skin of a fruit or vegetable is broken, don't eat it. Wash prepackaged salad mixes, even if the label says it's prewashed. Don't drink unpasteurized apple juice. (Which means don't drink most apple cider.)

★

question: Juice bars and health food places always offer smoothies. I've seen some made with protein powders; some offer "boosters" like ginseng, brewer's yeast, bee pollen, lecithin, calcium, wheat grass, spirulina, rice brans, and oat bran. Do the protein powders and boosters really do something for you? And what's spirulina anyway?

answer: Spirulina is a cultivated algae that has been called "the super food of the future" because it is an incredible protein source—it's said to contain all the essential amino acids, twice as much vitamin B_{12} as liver, and lots of other vitamins and minerals.

In general, according to nutritionists, these boosters and smoothies and fruit energy drinks will give you a quick burst of nutrition. Most likely, you'll be getting a bunch of vitamins, some calories for energy, maybe some protective value. They're thick, fun, fruity, but there's nothing super-powerful about them. And you can't just live on these drinks—you still need to get your nutrition in other ways.

Can you get *too much* of a good thing? Will you o.d. on bee pollen or wheat grass? According to nutritionist Michelle Daum, just the fact that ingredients are expensive makes it highly unlikely that you'll be getting a huge amount of any of these ingredients when you order a health drink at a restaurant or health food store. You're more likely to get too much if you go off to the health food store and buy the stuff yourself.

★

question: Were humans originally vegetarian?

answer: "Historically," say Virginia and Mark Messina in *The Vegetarian Way*, "fossil records show that throughout our evolution, humans and their ancestors definitely ate meat."

★

question: Why do beans make you fart?

answer: The problem with beans is that our bodies lack the enzyme to break down bean sugars. Bacteria (this sounds gross) feed on the sugar in our intestines in a natural fermentation process. It's this natural fermentation process that causes gas. There are two possible solutions: One is to introduce beans gradually into your diet. The other is to try a product like Beano, which contains the enzyme needed to digest bean sugars. Do these products really work? Nutritionists say that they seem to work for only about half their patients.

★

question: What about herbs? Is there anything I should know? Anything that would be good to take?

answer: Andrea Candee, a master herbalist in South Salem, New York, makes the argument that if you are adopting a healthy and holistic lifestyle, herbal remedies are far more organic and natural than synthetic pharmaceutical drugs. And when used properly, they don't have toxic side effects. Plus, they can help boost the body's immune system.

Instead of taking a one-a-day vitamin, she suggests taking Vitaherb, a 100 percent whole vitamin and mineral food made only from herbs. (Nature's Plus and Solgar are two others often recommended.) There are a few things herbs can help you with. For a healthy energy boost, Ms. Candee suggests Siberian ginseng, which you can get in liquid or tablet form in a health food store. And there are two energy drinks she's devised. The first one she calls Honegar. First, make a stock of one-half cup apple cider vinegar (get wood-aged cider vinegar from the health food store, not chemically aged) and one-half cup honey. (Don't refrigerate this.) Mix one to two tablespoons of this stock with a dropperful of cayenne tincture (it's like a liquid red pepper, also from the health food store) and add to a half glass of hot or cold water. You can take this three times a day.

Another energy drink calls for mixing one-half tablespoon of blackstrap molasses (regular dark molasses, which is high in minerals and iron) with one to two tablespoons of the Honegar stock plus a dropperful of the cayenne tincture in one-half cup of hot water. Ms. Candee notes that until you build up a tolerance, begin taking cayenne in drops.

Feel like you're coming down with something or have an upset stomach? A simple herbal solution might be fresh raw garlic. Garlic is another natural antibiotic, and just one or two cloves a day (mash them into potatoes or slice on toast) can cure an upset stomach.

You're under stress; you've got a sore throat; it's flu season and you're determined not to get sick. Protect yourself from any or all of the above with one of the most well-known herbal remedies, echinacea. If you start taking echinacea at the first sign of a cold or flu, you've got a good shot at having those symptoms disappear. The best way to take echinacea is in liquid extract form.

These are just a few herbal remedies—it's good to be open to various forms of health and nutrition as options or as alternative treatments. And for a vegetarian, these kinds of simple and natural solutions are definitely worth exploring. Needless to say, make sure you talk to a doctor or herbalist or health food store professional about dosages.

question: I can't figure out why they're called "veggie burgers" when they don't ever seem to be made with vegetables.

answer: The name veggie burger really just means that there is no animal fat used. Most veggie burgers are made from soy protein. Of course, there's black bean burgers, TVP burgers, mushroom burgers, etc.

question: Is there a connection between vegetarianism and eating disorders?

answer: Eating disorders like anorexia and bulimia, as you probably know, are rampant these days in America, especially with teenage girls. (Statistically, 95 percent of all people with eating disorders are women, according to the ADA's Food and Nutrition Guide.) But no one knows for sure whether there is one cause of these disorders or many. Theories abound. Is it because the ideal female shape in America today is almost unnaturally thin? Is it too many pictures of a gorgeous and skinny Kate Moss in the fashion magazines? Is it that there are so few things a teenager can really control, so that eating winds up being one of the few areas where he or she feels successfully in charge. Is it simply that there has never been a more difficult and stressful time to be a teenager and that food (love, nourishment, nurturing) somehow becomes an emotionally charged issue? Is it a way for teenagers, especially girls, to protest a culture that expects them to be perfect daughters, perfect students, perfect young women with perfect bodies? Is it a self-esteem issue—the less you think of yourself, the less you eat?

No one knows for sure, but there are a few things just about everyone agrees on. One, food isn't the primary problem—it's a symptom of whatever the real problem is. Two, eating disorders are extraordinarily complex. Three, there is a connection between them and vegetarianism. "Someone with an eating disorder will definitely cut out fat," says nutritionist Michelle Daum. "And often the first step in becoming anorexic is to cut out meat, which is high in fat." If you want to lose a lot of weight, but you don't want people to know, you can always use vegetarianism as an excuse. It's a great cover.

Ernst Schaefer, head of the Lipid Program at Tufts University School of Nutrition, has studied eating disorders for twenty years. "Most of America," Dr. Schaefer points out, "is overweight. But look at eating disorder clinics. They're filled with college-age women who don't get enough fat. These girls equate fat with meat. So they cut out meat. Plus, to them, vegetables equal health and strength, whereas meat equals immorality and weakness. So for them, vegetarianism becomes a weight-loss regime that's wrapped in a huge overlay of morality and philosophy." His sad conclusion: "While these well-intentioned vegetarian teenagers are saving the world, we are in danger of losing them." The bottom line is simple. While most teenage vegetarians probably won't develop an eating disorder, a high percentage of teens who have eating disorders or who are flirting with eating disorders will become vegetarians.

How do you know if you are at risk? If you are counting every fat gram; if you think you are grossly overweight even though everyone else says you're not; if you feel like the less you eat, the more powerful you become; if food and looks and weight are obsessions, then chances are you are developing a problem and ought to go talk to a nutritionist or doctor or psychotherapist or your parents. If you have a friend or roommate you are concerned about, suggest that they talk to someone. Just getting the problem out in the open is an important first step.

question: If you weren't getting enough protein, would you know it? Would you feel funny or weird?

answer: Unless you were acutely protein-deficient (which is incredibly rare), you wouldn't necessarily know.

question: If you have meat after you haven't had it for a very long time, will it make you sick?

answer: It shouldn't. But people who eat meat for the first time in months tend to say that they don't like the feeling—it makes them feel heavy or lethargic.

question: What does "virgin" olive oil mean? And what does "extra-virgin" mean?

answer: Terms like virgin and extra-virgin refer not to the age or the nutrient content or the dating experience of the oil, but simply refer to its acid content. Extra-virgin olive oil has less acid and a fruitier flavor than virgin olive oil.

★

question: Does soy milk last about the same amount of time in the refrigerator as regular milk?

answer: According to the Soyfoods Association of America (from *NT Times*, March 1998), the shelf life of soy milk and dairy milk are similar. If you refrigerate soy milk in its original container, it should stay good for about seven days. When it's going bad, soy milk lets off a funny odor and may turn thicker and clotted. Needless to say, don't drink it. FYI: soy milk that's packaged in those aseptic cartons can be stored in your pantry for several months. Once you open the carton, it requires refrigeration.

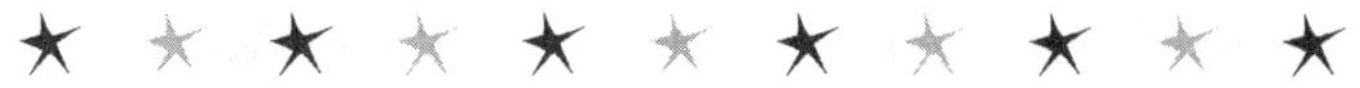

Afterword

I have a couple of observations after doing this book. I am convinced that the world is going to be a better place when today's teenagers take over. Today's *vegetarian* teenagers, that is.

As a group, you are thoughtful, caring, and articulate. You have a profound understanding of what really matters in the world. (It's a good thing I'm not a college admissions director—I would probably let all of you in.) And while so many of you are deeply committed to global issues like world hunger, world peace, and animal rights, you understand that change starts with small steps. You know that even the most mundane daily decision (recycling; using paper, not plastic; cleaning with nontoxic products; conserving water) can contribute to making the world a better place.

Saisha Uma-Michelle Grayson, a freshman at Sarah Lawrence College and lifelong vegetarian, puts it in perspective. She says, "I believe as the movement continues to grow, the impact we can have on our environment will also grow, and allow individuals to really have a positive influence on the world with every bite they take."

Making the world a better place bite by bite is a nice way to define what vegetarianism does. And as far as having a positive influence, I've observed that while you have been teaching yourself about vegetarianism, you have also been teaching us. All of us (your family, your friends, your classmates) wind up benefiting from your commitment and ideals and sacrifices. With the exception of some really awful parents you've told me about who disparage your decision to become vegetarian and won't help you in any way (and who could *definitely* benefit from reading this book), all the families I interviewed said that they feel they have learned a lot and changed a lot since you became a vegetarian.

They're eating a far healthier diet now. They're eating less meat or no meat at all. They're more aware of pesticides and good nutrition and natural foods. Aside from food issues, they have started to think more about issues that you've introduced: how to treat animals, how to protect the earth's resources, how to be a more compassionate person, how to live more simply and happily.

And thanks to you, they are more open to things like yoga and Buddhism and Tofutti and acupuncture and Chinese herbal teas and Fiona Apple (who is a vegan). I've almost forgiven Phoebe for making me take a beginners' tai chi class, after which she came out more mellow and centered and I came out with a neck sprain so pronounced that I am now going to physical therapy to cure it. More praise: there is an optimism and openness you have that most of us who are over forty (okay, fifty) can only envy. As far as the conventional wisdom that teenagers are passive and noncommittal, I can only say that passionate and involved and full of opinions seems much more accurate to me. As far as I can tell, the meek won't be inheriting the earth after all.

One more thing. You're remarkably patient. What I can't figure out is how a teenager who can't wait five minutes for a tape to rewind or twenty minutes for the pizza guy to ring the bell is willing to work on a cause so enormous that it could take a lifetime to achieve.

But bit by bit and bite by bite, you're making a difference. You should feel awfully good about yourselves. I know I felt good about writing this book.

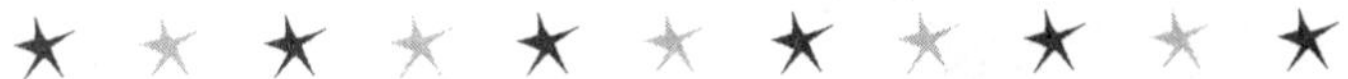

Resources

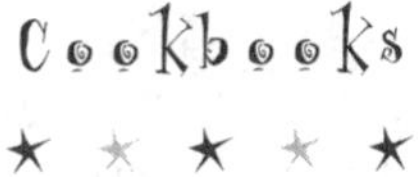

Cookbooks

Good & Cheap Vegetarian Dining in New York, by Arthur S. Brown and Barbara Holmes. City & Co., 1995.
Breezy, easy, helpful, hip.

1,000 Vegetarian Recipes, by Carol Gelles. Macmillan, 1996.
The 1997 winner of the IACP Julia Child Cookbook Award and James Beard Foundation Award, this is a comprehensive and well-conceived cookbook, with recipes appropriate for different types of vegetarians noted.

Feeding the Healthy Vegetarian Family, by Ken Haedrich. Bantam Books, 1998.
A wonderful cookbook devoted entirely to easy-to-cook vegetarian recipes the whole family will love.

The Moosewood Cookbook, by Mollie Katzen. Ten Speed Press, rev. 1992.
The updated version of the homey, healthy, satisfying bible.

Mollie Katzen's Vegetarian Heaven, by Mollie Katzen. Hyperion, 1997.
By the author of *The Enchanted Broccoli Forest,* an array of vegetarian recipes, with the emphasis on delicious and simple. Helpful comments and tips throughout.

Vegetarian Cooking for Everyone, by Deborah Madison. Broadway Books, 1997.

Longer than *Gone with the Wind* (742 pages!) but every bit as riveting. And much more delicious.

The Vegetarian Way, by Virginia Messina and Mark Messina. Three Rivers Press, 1996.

Although not a cookbook, this is a wonderfully comprehensive overview for the whole family. Well-researched and well-written. From the history of to the feeding of vegetarians, along with everything you might want to know about nutrition, health, diet, and philosophy. Special sections on teenagers and some recipes.

Moosewood Restaurant Low-Fat Favorites, by The Moosewood Collective. Clarkson Potter, 1996.

Delicious, creative, natural low-fat foods. As every Moosewood book, nice and inviting.

The New Laurel's Kitchen: A Handbook for Vegetarian Cookery and Nutrition, by Laurel Robertson, Carol Flinders, and Brian Ruppenthal. Ten Speed Press, 1986.

New Joy of Cooking, by Irma S. Rombauer, Marion Rombauer Becker, and Ethan Becker. Scribner, 1997.

The updated classic recipes for just about anything you could think of and lots that wouldn't occur to you! Not just vegetarian.

The New Vegetarian Epicure, by Anna Thomas. Alfred A. Knopf, 1996.

Ms. Thomas is cheerful, wise, balanced, a wonderful cook as well as a wonderful writer. If she ever had a fan club, I would be the president. This is a book to buy to use yourself or to give to your parents, so they will be inspired to cook wonderful things for all of you.

Vegetarian Times Complete Cookbook, by the editors of *Vegetarian Times*. MacMillan, 1995.

Over 600 vegetarian recipes, plus solid nutritional information. From the sublime (Summer Vegetable Risotto, Strawberry Angel Food Cake) to the ridiculous (Singapore Sling Seitan, Rice In A Lotus Leaf).

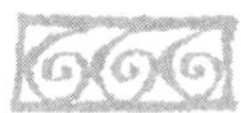

Nutrition Information

★ ★ ★ ★ ★

dial-a-nutritionist

This is a really great and unique service. If you want to find a registered dietician/nutritionist near where you live, someone who could make sure you're on a healthy vegetarian eating plan, the National Center for Nutrition and Dietetics has a hot line to call. To find an advisor in your area, call (800) 366–1655.

registered dieticians

For personalized answers to food and nutrition questions from registered dieticians, call (900) CALL-AN-RD (225–5267). Hours are 9:00 A.M. to 4:00 P.M., Central time, Monday through Friday. Calls are $1.95 for the first minute and $0.95 for each additional minute.

vegetarian nutrition

Quarterly newsletter and fact sheets from the American Dietetic Association. This group was founded in 1990 to provide objective information about food and nutrition. It's located in Chicago and, with seventy thousand members, is the nation's largest organization of food and nutrition professionals. There is a lot this group does and some great resources they provide. Their Vegetarian Nutrition Practice Group publishes the quarterly newsletter *Issues in Vegetarian Dietetics.* Then, free of charge, via the newsletter, they distribute new fact sheets. For information, call the ADA at (312) 899–0040.

the vegan foundation

P.O. Box 1933
Cupertino, California 95015–1933
http://www.vegan.com
Founded by Erik Marcus, author of the book *Vegan, The New Ethics of Eating* (McBooks, 1998), this fairly new organization promotes vegan diets and gives the latest vegan news and resources, plus vegan recipes.

the vegetarian starter kit

A basic and sensible diet/nutrition pamphlet for beginners published by the Physicians Committee for Responsible Medicine. Write to them at 5100 Wisconsin Avenue NW, Suite 404, Washington, DC 20016 or call (202) 686–2210.

Gardening

★ ★ ★ ★ ★

Grow your own, or make your parents do it for you! To get started, send for some free garden seed catalogs.

W. Atlee Burpee
300 Park Avenue
Warminster, PA 18974
(800) 888–1447

The Cook's Garden
Box 535
Londonderry, VT 05148
(800) 457–9703

Park Seed
Cokesbury Road
Greenwood, SC 29647
(800) 845–3369

Seeds of Change
Box 15700
Santa Fe, NM 87506
(800) 957–3337

Shepherd's Garden Seeds
30 Irene Street
Torrington, CT 06790
(860) 482–3638

Sproutpeople
E-mail: sprouts@sproutpeople.com
Or write to: Sproutpeople
225 Main Street
Gays Mills, WI 54631

This small company in Wisconsin grows and sells crunchy, healthy sprouts. Everything from alfalfa to sunflower to the hottest new star on the sprout horizon, broccoli, which was recently found to have anti-cancer properties. Grow your own (all you need is a windowsill) by ordering a sprout kit (from *Health* magazine, April 1998).

Mail Order and Markets

★ ★ ★ ★ ★

walnut acres—organic farms

"A Catalogue of Whole Food for Healthy Living Direct from America's Original Organic Farm." For catalog call (800) 344–9025, Monday to Friday between 8:00 A.M. and 4:00 P.M., Eastern time. Walnut Acres, in Penns Creek, Pennsylvania, isn't a vegetarian catalog, but their non-meat offerings are great: fresh, homemade granolas (raspberry crunch, toasted hazelnut); organic three-bean vegetarian chili; peanut honey sesame spread; cranberry nectar—the highest quality, best, and freshest.

the national farmers' market directory

There are twenty-five hundred farmers' markets in the United States. Look up the one nearest you in *The National Farmers' Market Directory.* For a free copy, write the U.S. Department of Agriculture, Box 96456, Room 2642 South, Washington, DC 20090. Or call (202) 720–8317.

phipps country beans

You can order organic beans from this small, dedicated family farm. They use no sprays, harvest mostly by hand, and sell everything from well-known varieties like pinto and lima to heirloom varieties that are fun to try. Write to P.O. Box 349, Pescadero, CA 94060. Or call (800) 279–0889 or (650) 879–0787. You can even send a fax: (650) 879–1662.

american spoon foods

Renowned American chef Larry Forgione is the guru who thought of gathering the freshest, ripest tastes in America, mostly from northern Michigan, and forming a mail-order business. The catalog includes everything from Michigan maple syrup to dried red tart cherries to Wild Thimbleberry jam. (If I sound a little extra gung-ho on Larry, it's because I'm a big fan and helped write his award-winning cookbook, *An American Place.*) Write: P.O. Box 566, Petoskey, MI 49770–0566; call: (888) 735–6700 or (616) 347–9030; or fax: (616) 347–2512. Larry even has a Web site: www.spoon.coe-mail:information@spoon.com.

Good Web Sites

★ ★ ★ ★ ★

"vegetarian youth online"

http://www.geocities.com/RainForest/Vines/4482/

Their description of themselves: "a grassroots, web-based organization run entirely by, and for, youth who support compassionate, healthy, globally-aware, vegetarian/vegan living."

"vegan action"

http://www.vegan.org

"vegan outreach"

http://www.vegsource.com/vo/index/html

"veg source"

http://www.vegsource.com/

"farm sanctuary web page"

http://www.farmsanctuary.org

"veggies unite!"

http://vegweb.com

"vegetarian resource group"

http://www.vrg.org/

"vegetarian pages"

http://www.veg.org/veg/

one-stop online nutrition shopping

What a great idea from Tufts University. There are now so many food and nutrition Web sites that it's both hard to keep up and hard to figure out who to trust for the most accurate information. So Tufts, which has one of the best schools of nutrition in the country, came up with Nutrition Navigator (http://www.navigator.tufts.edu), the first site to review and rate nutrition sites.

Veg on the Edge

★ ★ ★ ★ ★

bow wow distributors

Mail-order pet foods. "The finest Vegan and Vegetarian pet foods, the most humane meat based foods, as well as an extensive line of alternative therapies." Not only can you do the right thing by your cat or dog, Bow Wow promises that they can customize any order. More good news: all their biscuits are available with organically grown ingredients upon request. Write: 13B Lucon Drive, Deer Park, NY 11729. Call: (800) 326–0230.

tofurky

One more thing to give thanks for: Turtle Island Foods in Hood River, Oregon, has created Tofurky, a meatless feast. The main course is a prebaked seasoned tofu "roast." It comes with tempeh drumsticks, golden mushroom gravy, and wild rice. The entire meal, which serves four, is rich in protein and fiber and very low in saturated fat. Tofurky is in natural health food stores, or order it for next-day delivery by calling (800) 863–8759. (From *Bon Appetit,* October 1997.)

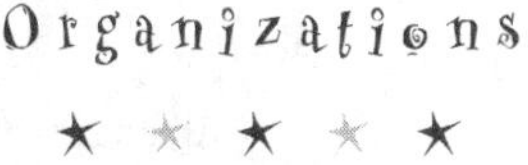

earthsave international

An environmental organization founded by John Robbins *(Diet for a New America)* that is dedicated to creating a better world and encourages "the benefits of healthy and life-sustaining food choices" as a means to that end. Write: 600 Distillery Commons, Suite 200, Louisville, KY 40206-1922. Call: (502) 589-7676 or (800) DNA-DOIT.

yes! youth for environmental sanity

A teen off-shoot of EarthSave, founded by John Robbins's son Ocean. This environmental activist group conducts speaking tours and workshops, writes books and action guides, and runs a summer camp program. Write: 420 Bronco Road, Soquel, CA 95073. Call: (408) 662–0793. Fax: (408) 662–0797. Web site: http://www.yesworld.org.

vegetarian resource group

These very nice people, who run one of the largest and most respected national organizations, will send you helpful vegetarian information, including guides to teen nutrition. There's also a special student membership and a vegan teen chat list online guide. Write: P.O. Box 1343, Baltimore, MD 21203. Call: (410) 366–VEGE. Web site: http://www.veg.org.

VRG is the single best resource I had researching this book. You can count on them for everything from the most helpful attitude to the most up-to-date advice. In case you're in Baltimore at Thanksgiving, they give an annual community vegetarian dinner that is much loved.

other organizations

American Vegan Society
501 Old Harding Highway
Malaga, NJ 08328
(609) 694–2887

Farm Sanctuary
P.O. Box 150
Watkins Glen, NY 14891–0150
(607) 583–2225

The Fund for Animals
850 Sligo Avenue
Suite LL2
Silver Spring, MD 20901
(301) 585–2591

North American Vegetarian Society
P.O. Box 72
Dolgeville, NY 13329
(518) 568–7970

People for the Ethical Treatment of Animals
P.O. Box 42516
Washington, DC 20015
(202) 726–0156

Humane Society of the United States
2100 L Street, NW
Washington, DC 20037
(202) 452–1100

Farm Animal Reform Movement
P.O. Box 70123
Washington, DC 20088
(301) 530–1737

American Friends Service Committee
1501 Cherry Street
Philadelphia, PA 19102
(215) 241–7000

Oxfam America
115 Broadway
Boston, MA 02116
(617) 482–1211

Greenpeace
1611 Connecticut Avenue, NW
Washington, DC 20009
(202) 462–1177

Friends of the Earth
530 Seventh Street, SE
Washington, DC 20003
(202) 543–4312

Greenhouse Crisis Foundation
1130 Seventeenth Street, NW
Suite 630
Washington, DC 20036
(202) 466–2823

International Vegetarian Society
A year-old group that embraces the positive aspects of vegetarianism and that bills itself as "a consumer report for people who want good, solid answers on new discoveries in diet and lifestyles." The executive director of this Colorado Springs group is Maelu Fleek. Call: 408–415–1081 or fax: 408–462–6970.

Restaurants

★ ★ ★ ★ ★

One of the most comprehensive guides to vegetarian restaurants in North America is the *Vegetarian Journal's Guide to Natural Foods Restaurants in the United States and Canada,* available from the Vegetarian Resource Group (410–366–VEGE) for $14.00. For overseas, there's the *European Vegetarian Guide: Restaurants and Hotels,* published in Germany but also available through the VRG for $16.00 (in English translation). Online, the "World Guide to Vegetarianism" Web site (www.veg.org/veg/Guide/) lists restaurants by country, state, city, and vegetarian category. *Condé Nast Traveler* (February 1997) wisely states that restaurant information can get stale quickly, so call ahead.

Atlanta

Café Sunflower (5975 Roswell Road, Suite 353, 404–256–1675; Asian, European, and Southwestern influences)

Soul Vegetarian (879 Abernathy Boulevard SW, 404–752–5194; African)

Soul Vegetarian II (North Highland Avenue, just south of Ponce de Leon and Virginia Highlands; African)

Austin

West Lynn Cafe (1110 West Lynn Street; highly recommended; 512–482–0950)

Mr. Natural (1901 East First Street; recommended by the Austin Vegetarian Society; 512–477–5228)

Baltimore

Margaret's Café (909 Fell Street, 410–276–5605)

Thai (3316–18 Greenmount Avenue, 410–889–7303)

Boston Area

Centre Street Café (597 Centre Street, Jamaica Plain, 617–524–9217; "Jamaican Plain Eclectic")

Country Life Vegetarian (200 High Street, Boston, 617–951–2534; all-you-can-eat natural food)

Milk Street Cafe (Post Office Square, Boston, 617–542–3663; and 50 Milk Street, Boston)

Chicago Area

Heartland Cafe (7000 North Glenwood Avenue, 773–465–8005)

Blind Faith Café (525 Dempster Street, Evanston, 847–328–6875)

Chicago Diner (3411 Halsted Street, 773–935–6696; offers vegan, macrobiotic)

Chowpatti Vegetarian (1035 South Arlington Heights Road, 847–640–9554)

Colorado

The Harvest (1738 Pearl Street, Boulder, 303–449–6223; 430 South Colorado Boulevard, Denver, 303–399–6652; and 7730 East Belleview Avenue, Greenwood Village, 303–779–4111)

Himalayas (2010 Fourteenth Street, Boulder, 303–442–3230; vegetarian and Indian)

Dallas

Anand Bhavan Vegetarian (115 Spring Valley Village, 972–783–4353; Indian)

Dream Cafe (Quadrangle, 2800 Routh Street, 214–954–0486; and 1133 North Zang Boulevard; 214–943–6448; "eclectic")

Macro Broccoli (Camelto Shopping Center, 580 West Arapaho Road, Suite 406, Richardson, 972–437–1985; macrobiotic)

Whole Foods Market/Cafe Juice Bar (Whole Foods Market, 2218 Greenville Avenue, 214–828–0052)

Fort Worth

Sunflower Cafe (5817 Curzon Avenue, 817–738–5454)

Fort Lauderdale

Bread of Life (2388 North Federal Highway, 954–565–7423)

Kansas City, MO

Bluebird at City Garden (1700 Summit Street, 816–221–7559; coffee-house feel)

Los Angeles Area

Inn of the Seventh Ray (128 Old Topanga Canyon Road, Topanga, 310–455–1311; homemade health foods, etc.)

Mother's Market & Kitchen (225 East Seventeenth Street, Costa Mesa, 714–631–4741; and Newland Shopping Center, 19770 Beach Boulevard, Huntington Beach, 714–963–6667)

Ranch House (South Lomita Avenue, Ojal, 805–646–2360)

The Source (8301 Sunset Boulevard, West Hollywood, 213–656–6388)

Follow Your Heart (21825 Sherman Way, 818–348–3240; vegan friendly)

Miami

Tulasi (12260 Southwest Eighth Street, 305–554–8989; Indian, international, salad bar)

New Orleans

Back to the Garden (YMCA Hotel, 920 Saint Charles Avenue, 504–522–8792)

All Natural Foods (5517 Magazine Street, 504–891–2651)

New York City

Angelica Kitchen (300 East Twelfth Street, 212–228–2909; Phoebe's favorite restaurant in the whole world. This is the natural foods restaurant others aspire to: the highest standards, the most reasonable prices, a reverence for quality ingredients)

Zen Palate (663 Ninth Avenue, 212–582–1669; and 34 Union Square East, 212–614–9345)

Rice (227 Mott Street, 212–226–5775; only in New York, an all rice restaurant—the place is tiny but the menu is expansive—everything from sticky rice to vegetarian meatballs)

Blanche's Organic Café (East Forty-fourth between Fifth and Madison, 212–599–3445; and Seventy-first and Lexington 212–717–1923; hip and delicious and friendly; Phoebe's other favorite; really good chocolate chip cookies and scrambled tofu)

Drovers Tap Room (also Home and Home Away From Home Takeout; 9 Jones Street, 212–627–1182; homey and welcoming food experience; not veg, but lots of good vegetarian food; brought to you by David Page and Barbara Shinn, both sticklers for freshness and down-home taste)

North Carolina

The Laughing Seed Cafe (40 Wall Street, Asheville, 704–252–3445)

Philadelphia

Harmony Vegetarian (135 North Ninth Street, Chinatown, 215–627–4520; good for vegans)

Singapore (Race Street between Tenth and Eleventh, Chinatown, 215–922–3288; substitutions for all meat)

Basic 4 Vegetarian Food Bar (Reading Terminal Market, Twelfth and Filbert Streets, 215–440–0991)

San Diego Area

Jyoti Blhange (3351 Adams Avenue, 619–282–4116)

Kung Food Vegetarian (2949 Fifth Avenue, 619–298–7330)

Monsoon (Village Hillcrest Shopping Center, 3975 Fifth Avenue, 619–298–3155; strong Indian emphasis)

San Francisco Area

Millennium Restaurant (Abigail Hotel, 246 McAllister Street, 415–487–9800)

Raw Experience Foods (1224 Ninth Avenue, 415–665–6519; all the organic foods are served raw!)

Valentine's Cafe (1793 Church Street, 415–285–2257; international theme, "artsy Mission Vegetarian")

Long Life Vegi House (2129 University Avenue, Berkeley, 510–845–6072)

Utah

Oasis Cafe (151 South 500 East, Salt Lake City, 801–322–0404; bistro-coffeehouse setting)

Vermont

Five Spice Café (175 Church Street, Burlington, 802–864–4045; best Pan-Asian food in the area; a favorite with University of Vermont students; great vegetable dim sum)

Washington, DC, Area

Delight of the Garden (2616 Georgia Avenue NW, Washington, DC, 202–319–8747; only raw vegan of its kind in the DC area)

Planet X (7422 Baltimore Avenue, College Park, MD, 301–779–8451; " '90s food meets '60s coffeehouse chic")

Udupi Palace (1325 University Boulevard, Langey Park, MD, 301–434–1431; southern Indian)

Himalayan Grill (1805 Eighteenth Street, NW, Washington, DC, 202–986–5124; "suitable for casual or romantic dining")

Vegetable Garden (11618 Rockville Pike, Rockville, MD, 301–468–9301; alternative Chinese)

Wisconsin

Beans & Barley (1901 East North Avenue, Milwaukee, 414–278–7878)

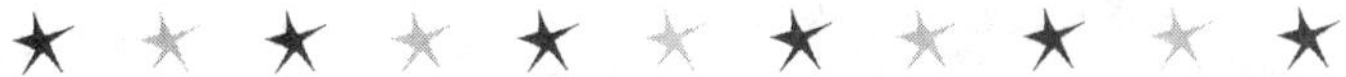

General Index

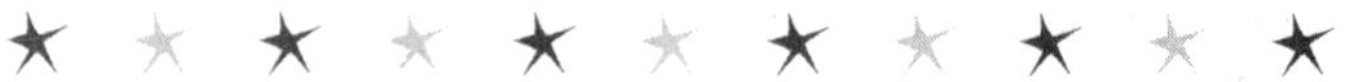

Recipe Index

C

D

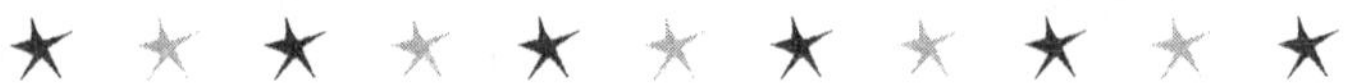

Stephanie Pierson lives with her family in South Salem, New York. She has two daughters, two dogs, two cats, and one husband. She is the author of the book, *Because I'm the Mother, That's Why!* a lighthearted look at modern motherhood. She has written two cookbooks and also writes food and lifestyle articles for magazines like *Metropolitan Home, Saveur,* and *McCalls.*